How to Teach in Clinical Settings

How to Teach in Clinical Settings

Mary Seabrook

Medical Education Consultant
Former Senior Lecturer in Medical Education
King's College London School of Medicine
London, UK

⊛WILEY-BLACKWELL

A John Wiley & Sons, Ltd., Publication

This edition first published 2014 © 2014 by John Wiley & Sons, Ltd.

Registered office: John Wiley & Sons, Ltd, The Atrium, Southern Gate, Chichester, West Sussex, PO19 8SQ, UK

Editorial offices: 9600 Garsington Road, Oxford, OX4 2DQ, UK
The Atrium, Southern Gate, Chichester, West Sussex, PO19 8SQ, UK
111 River Street, Hoboken, NJ 07030-5774, USA

For details of our global editorial offices, for customer services and for information about how to apply for permission to reuse the copyright material in this book please see our website at www.wiley.com/wiley-blackwell

Library of Congress Cataloging-in-Publication Data
Seabrook, Mary, 1960- author.
  How to teach in clinical settings / Mary Seabrook.
      p. ; cm.
  Includes bibliographical references and index.
  ISBN 978-1-118-62093-9 (pbk.)
  I. Title.
  [DNLM: 1. Education, Medical. 2. Teaching – methods. 3. Clinical Competence. 4. Learning.
W 18]
  R834.5
  610.71 – dc23

                                                              2013029215

A catalogue record for this book is available from the British Library.

Wiley also publishes its books in a variety of electronic formats. Some content that appears in print may not be available in electronic books.

Cover design by Meaden Creative

Typeset in 9.5/12 pt Minion by Laserwords Private Limited, Chennai, India
Printed and bound in Malaysia by Vivar Printing Sdn Bhd

1   2014

Contents

Acknowledgements, ix
Introduction, xi

Chapter 1 Creating an effective learning environment, 1
Practical ways to create an environment conducive to
learning, 4
Design of clinical placements, 6
Continuity between learners, teachers and patients, 8
Teaching and learning resources, 9
The teaching climate, 9
What makes a good clinical teacher?, 10
Involving patients in teaching, 11
Involving other disciplines in teaching, 13
Some principles of effective clinical teaching, 15
Useful strategies for clinical teaching, 15
Five tips for clinical teaching which do not take time or
money, 17
References, 17

Chapter 2 Teaching in clinical contexts, 19
Teaching on ward rounds, 19
General principles, 19
Useful strategies, 21
What you teach unwittingly, 23
The psychiatric ward round, 25
Handover meetings, board rounds and bench rounds, 26
Bedside teaching, 29
Preparation, 29
Structure for bedside teaching, 30
Feedback at the bedside, 34
Examination practice at the bedside, 36

Teaching in clinics, 38
General principles, 38
Supervising trainees in parallel clinics, 40
Effective questioning on presented cases, 41
Seeing the patient together, 42
Supervising students or trainees who are supernumerary, 43
Teaching in the Accident and Emergency department, 46
Teaching the interpretation of images/specimens, 47
Teaching in theatre, 49
General principles, 50
Useful strategies, 50
Teaching practical skills, 56
On-call/remote teaching, 60
Teaching patients, 62
Teaching other disciplines, 64
Further reading on clinical teaching, 65
References, 66

Chapter 3 Workplace-based assessment and feedback, 67
The workplace-based assessments/supervised learning
events, 67
Using the tools effectively, 69
Case-based discussion, 71
The mini-clinical evaluation exercise (Mini-ACE in
psychiatry), 73
Directly observed procedural skills, 75
Multi-source feedback (MSF), 77
Teaching observation tools, 79
Giving feedback, 81
Giving negative feedback, 81
General principles of feedback, 82
Useful strategies for giving feedback, 82
Feedback models and structures, 85
Further reading on assessment and feedback, 89
References, 90

Chapter 4 Common problems in clinical teaching, 91
Balancing teaching and service demands, 91
Pitching teaching at the right level , 94
Dealing with complaints and clinical incidents, 96

Ad hoc teaching, 100
Teaching people at different levels together, 101
Teaching older or more experienced colleagues, 103
Engaging the quiet or reluctant learner, 104
The difficult consultation, 106
Teaching multiple students, 107
Teaching trainees with no interest in your speciality, 108
References, 109

Chapter 5 Next steps, 110
Developing as a teacher, 110
Evaluating your teaching, 111
Useful resources, 115

Appendix Glossary of assessment tools, 118

Index, 119

Acknowledgements

Thanks to the following people who have assisted with providing examples, reviewing draft material or other support:
Amrit Sachar, Stephanie Strachan, Catherine Bryant, Adam Chambers, Fahmida Chowdhury, Nicholas Culshaw, Yaya Egberongbe, Jeban Ganesalingham, Richard Gummer, Deepak Joshi, Diana Kelly, TJ Lasoye, Mary Lawson, Heidi Lempp, Thomas Lloyd, Camilla Kingdon, Deepti Radia, Catherine Scrymgeour-Wedderburn, Alex Seabrook, Matt Staff, Nishanthan Srikanatha, Rosalinde Tilley and Alan Taylor. I am also indebted to all the doctors and colleagues I have worked with over the years.
Special thanks to Helen Graham and Rachael Morris-Jones for inspiring me.

Introduction

Traditionally, learning to become a doctor has been an apprenticeship, with students and junior doctors working alongside practising clinicians and gradually taking on more responsibility for patient care. In recent years, the nature of the apprenticeship has changed: in many places, the master–apprentice relationship has become less prominent and junior doctors now work within wider teams of colleagues. At the same time, there has been an increased formalisation of training with the development of curricula that specify what is expected at each stage. There has also been more emphasis on providing regular, structured teaching, which tends to take place away from immediate clinical demands.

Nothing, however, can replace the centrality of 'on-the-job' learning because assessing and managing patients requires so much more than can ever be taught in a lecture theatre. Over 100 years ago, William Osler said that

To study the phenomena of disease without books is to sail an uncharted sea, while to study books without patients is not to go to sea at all [1].

In a clinical environment, people, often unconsciously, take in the sights, smells, sounds, the way in which the team works and decisions are made – multiple facets and subtle nuances of practice that can only be learnt on the job. Doctors often call this 'learning by osmosis' and, although much can be learnt in this way, learning can be greatly enhanced by good supervision.

Individual supervisors can make a real difference, but face conflicting demands as clinical environments have become increasingly pressurised. Greater bureaucracy, busier clinics, less time with patients and targets focused on clinical work rather than education, all make finding time for teaching challenging.

This book aims to help medical teachers/supervisors at whatever stage – from students to consultants – to explore different ways in which to help others learn. It is designed primarily as a practical manual, providing examples of hands-on strategies that can be used in daily supervision and teaching. These have been gathered from first-hand observation or reports of effective teaching provided by students and doctors. The content is underpinned by educational theory and evidence, but references and theoretical explanations are kept to a minimum as there are many existing books that cover this material (see Further Reading sections).

The book is divided into five chapters:
1. Creating an effective learning environment.
2. Teaching in clinical contexts: strategies suitable for teaching during routine clinical work and for teaching patients and other disciplines.
3. Workplace-based assessment and feedback: effective ways to use the current tools.
4. Common problems in clinical teaching: guidance on issues such as teaching multiple students and pitching teaching at the right level.
5. Next steps: suggestions for further developing your teaching.

Not everything will be relevant to everyone, but there should be something for all. Some suggestions may seem idealistic, but the contexts in which doctors teach vary enormously, so select what is appropriate to your context. The book was written for doctors in hospital and community trusts, but some sections may also be relevant to general practitioners or other disciplines.

Some ideas or information relate specifically to *students* (undergraduates), others to *trainees* (postgraduates) and some to both (*learners*). *Teachers* and *supervisors* refer to those in a teaching or supervisory role, whatever their level of seniority.

Each chapter has a number of sections containing some or all of the following:

General principles of teaching relevant to particular clinical settings.

Useful strategies: drawn from good practice observed by the author or described by medical students or doctors.

Vignettes: practical examples of teaching and learning, chosen to illustrate specific points.

Quotes: from famous people about education.

Teachers' and learners' comments: views from the shop floor (sometimes paraphrased).

Challenges and thinking points: designed to help you explore key issues and apply ideas to your own teaching.

Discussions: commenting on the challenges and thinking points.

Theories of learning: a few theories of particular relevance are included.

Further reading: a personal selection of recommended articles and books. This book is designed as a resource for teachers to dip into for ideas and inspiration – hopefully helping to expand their repertoire of approaches and understanding of effective teaching and learning.

Reference

[1] Osler W. *Aequanimitas: with other addresses to medical students, nurses and practitioners of medicine*. Philadelphia: P. Blakiston's Son & Co; 1906. p. 220.

Chapter 1 **Creating an effective learning environment**

The clinical environment can be an exciting and, at the same time, daunting place in which to learn. Students entering clinical placements have to adjust to learning in a work environment, where, unlike at school or college, their learning is not the organisation's primary goal. They are usually enthused by the prospect of clinical work but feel that they lack a genuine role or place in the team. They may need help to learn how to gain access to patients and find learning opportunities.

So what determines how much people learn in workplace settings such as hospitals and general practices?

A study of learning at work found three main factors (Table 1.1).

Depending on your role, you may be able to impact on different areas. Most people find it quite easy to teach a motivated, competent and appropriately confident student or trainee. However, what if a trainee appears uninterested or lacking basic clinical skills? Someone in a pastoral role such as an educational supervisor or a personal tutor could address areas such as a learner's confidence and motivation. They might also help learners to set goals for developing their clinical skills, with teachers at all levels providing opportunities for practice and feedback.

Someone with a more strategic role such as a course organiser or training programme director may have some influence on the broader context, for example, ensuring that learners have adequate time for private study in their timetable.

Those supervising learners on a daily basis (often students or trainees at the next level up) will probably have most influence on their immediate conditions of work, such as the climate for learning and the type of work in which they are engaged. These aspects (which are addressed in the next

How to Teach in Clinical Settings, First Edition. Mary Seabrook.
© 2014 John Wiley & Sons, Ltd. Published 2014 by John Wiley & Sons, Ltd.

Table 1.1 Main factors affecting learning at work [1].

Factor	Examples
1. Characteristics of the learner	Confidence, motivation, capability, prior knowledge (This is probably the most important factor, accounting for about 50% of variance in learning.) [2]
2. The immediate work culture	Level of challenge and responsibility, quality of supervision/management, emotional support, learning climate, pressures and priorities
3. The broader context	The career structure, appraisal systems, working hours, training policies

two sections) are important, and sometimes underestimated, although not by Albert Einstein, who is reported to have said

> I never teach my pupils; I only attempt to provide the conditions in which they can learn [3].

Thinking point

Can you remember your early clinical placements as a student or newly qualified doctor? What were your first impressions? What messages did you receive about how easy or difficult learning would be? What, if anything, would have made you feel more ready and able to learn? What do you think is the optimum climate for learning?

Discussion

Most doctors will have had mixed experiences. Learners report positive aspects such as supportive teams, effective, approachable teachers and constructive feedback, and difficulties such as unstable or incomplete teams, lack of patient continuity and teaching by humiliation [4–6]. Views on the ideal learning climate also vary, both individually and between specialties. Some favour a supportive environment. Others believe that exposing learners' deficiencies publicly is necessary to protect patients, maintain standards and prepare doctors for the demands of their working lives [7]. Evidence from relevant research studies follows.

Factors identified by medical students as influencing the effectiveness of placements at a large teaching hospital are shown in Table 1.2. Trainees mention similar helpful characteristics: a study of resident medical officers in Australia identified eight elements of a placement contributing to professional development (Table 1.3).

Both studies highlight the importance of clear expectations, opportunities for practical experience and the exercise of responsibility. They also agree on the need for a social climate in which learners feel accepted and valued.

Table 1.2 Medical students' experiences of clinical placements [6]

What students found helpful	What students found difficult
Feeling valued within the team	Feeling in the way
Being made to feel useful	Being ignored
Having a forum to discuss their ideas where they will not be laughed at	Being talked over and not having things explained to them
Friendly, accessible and approachable staff	Not being able to contribute to patient care
Staff who want to teach	A pattern of teachers being late or cancelling planned teaching
Lots of practical experience and exposure	Hanging around waiting for opportunities
Doctors being interested in what they are doing	Lack of induction – learning by getting things wrong
Expectations being made explicit	

Table 1.3 Elements of the clinical environment perceived by trainees as contributing to learning.

Element	Description
Autonomy	Responsibility for patient care
Supervision	Guidance and direction from senior medical colleagues
Social support	Being accepted, recognised and valued within the team
Workload	Balance between service and professional development
Role clarity	Clarity of expectations about what should be done and achieved
Variety	Diversification of the work
Orientation to learning and teaching	Emphasis on learning and development and availability of learning activities
Orientation to general practice	Attention given to learning requirements relevant to general practice

Adapted from [8] with permission from Taylor & Francis Ltd.

These findings are supported by a major review of educational research which found that expert teachers respect students, both as learners and as people, showing care and commitment for them [2]. The optimal educational climate is described as one '*where error is welcomed, where student questioning is high, where engagement is the norm*' [2].

In a clinical context, error would not be *welcomed*, but it is safer for patients if the climate is sufficiently open that learners are not afraid to ask questions or admit mistakes or weaknesses [9,10]. It is easy for senior doctors to forget how scary they can seem to those lower down the hierarchy! At the same time, a culture of high expectations is important, with teachers demonstrating high standards themselves and expecting the same of their learners [11].

Practical ways to create an environment conducive to learning

Aim for a combination of challenge (setting goals and tasks which are demanding but achievable) and support (providing advice, encouragement and feedback to enable goals to be met). Practical things you can do include the following.

Before students/trainees arrive
- Send a welcome letter/e-mail to let them know where and when to come and what to bring.
- You may want to suggest how they could prepare for their placement, for example, relevant reading.

On arrival
Make them feel welcome/part of the team:
- remember and use their name;
- show a personal interest, for example, finding out more about their previous jobs, travel to work, spare time activities;
- find somewhere that they can meet, put things, access resources.

Orientate them (Box 1.1):
- introduce them to key colleagues;
- provide a proper induction, including written information;
- show them where to find and how to use relevant equipment or protocols;
- advise them how to learn – for example, what questions to ask themselves about patients, what to do when clinicians are late or do not arrive for teaching, how to focus their reading;
- direct them to relevant Intranet pages – ask current/past students to develop a list of useful resources which can be continuously modified by new trainees;
- tell them good times to contact you and how to do so (Box 1.2).

Box 1.1 Planning for new trainees

Mr. Jones, a colorectal surgeon, always takes a week's holiday in the first week of August. This means that there are fewer inpatients, so it is a quieter period during which the new trainees can become acquainted with the wards and get to know their colleagues before the normal busy routine resumes.

Conversely Dr. Payne in A&E ensures that there is good consultant cover during the first week of a new group of trainees. This allows them to provide induction training and close supervision of trainees during their early days in post.

Box 1.2 Addressing a problem

A consultant received feedback that she was not considered accessible by junior colleagues. She decided to nominate 1 hour a week where she would be in her office and juniors were invited to drop in with any queries. This worked well for her and the trainees.

Clarify expectations:
- explain what they can expect from the rotation, and perhaps what they cannot;
- explain the behaviour and standards you expect from them (e.g. dress code, punctuality, when/how to report back on patients);
- negotiate specific learning objectives;
- ask trainees/students from a previous rotation to advise them on working in the team – they will tend to tap into the things that newcomers want to know.

During the placement
- introduce them to patients from whom they can learn;
- be aware of curricular requirements (Box 1.3);
- provide feedback and open discussion of cases in which they are involved;
- periodically check how they are getting on and any problems they are having;
- provide a structured teaching programme covering common diseases/ problems, with arrangements to cover clinical duties so that they can attend;
- give sufficient time for ward-based teaching;

Box 1.3 A novel approach to sign-offs?

A group of students met a consultant for bedside teaching. The consultant took all their log books, immediately ticked and signed all the relevant sections and then told them that anyone who wanted to could now leave. No one did.

Whilst this method is not recommended, by signing everyone off, the consultant diverted the students' attention away from their log books, and allowed them to focus on the learning. How else could you achieve this?

- include them in team social events;
- adapt your teaching to the differing levels and needs of individuals;
- recognise when they are struggling and provide support – personal or professional.

These strategies should help newcomers to settle in and start to learn quickly and effectively.

Design of clinical placements

This section is most relevant to teachers who are in a position to influence students' or trainees' timetables.

Most learning at work arises not from formal teaching but from the challenges posed by the work itself, such as solving problems and interacting with colleagues and patients [1].

Thinking point

Does this reflect your experience? Think of times when you learnt a lot and those when you learnt less. What factors enhanced/inhibited learning?

Discussion

Many doctors remember being on call as a prime time for learning because they had to take decisions and bear the consequences, albeit sometimes in difficult and stressful circumstances. Acting up for more senior colleagues also provides a sharp learning curve.

In an apprenticeship, the development of expertise depends primarily on the quantity and quality of learning opportunities inherent in the work. So the type and scope of work in which learners are engaged and the level of responsibility they assume are important.

Learners will naturally increase their expertise fastest in relation to the conditions and stages of care that they see most commonly. So a useful question to ask about any placement is

- Are the types and numbers of patients to which trainees are exposed, and the stages at which they are involved, in line with the objectives of their training?

Placements are not always well matched to the stage of the learner, for example,

- Students or junior trainees are sometimes placed in highly specialised teams – opportunities which may be better suited to specialist trainees.
- Trainees may be busy on the wards, learning a lot about day-to-day management of patients but missing opportunities to learn about diagnosis, surgical interventions or long-term management.

These situations often occur because of service pressures, difficulty in finding placements or the increasingly specialised nature of health care. It is often argued that trainees will learn generic skills such as history taking or examination skills, although the evidence suggests that such skills are not easily transferable from one situation to another [12]. For example, taking histories from patients with anorexia does not prepare you for taking histories from patients with anaemia or even with another psychiatric condition because they rely on different underpinning knowledge bases.

Thinking point

Consider the timetable that your trainees work. Where are their learning opportunities focused? Are they seeing enough patients? Is the case mix appropriate? Are they seeing patients at different stages of care? Are they learning the skills and knowledge they need?

Where are the gaps? What other experiences would they benefit from? How could you improve their exposure?

Consider the same questions for your students.

Discussion

Ways in which some supervisors have addressed a mismatch between the timetable and learners' objectives include

- alerting learners to interesting patients whom they would otherwise miss;
- facilitating attendance at clinics or theatre sessions;
- organising swaps between trainees working in different contexts;

- considering progression during the placement, for example, getting trainees to
  - attend extra or different clinics/lists as they progress,
  - take on extra roles or responsibilities;
- encouraging the use of study days to enhance clinical exposure (e.g. through out of placement attachments), not just for courses or private study;
- focusing formal teaching on recognised gaps in clinical exposure.

Continuity between learners, teachers and patients

In recent years, continuity between trainees and patients has been reduced by shorter hospital stays and greater movement of patients between clinical teams. Thus, trainees are often unaware of the outcomes of their decisions. Similarly, continuity between trainee and supervisor/team has been reduced by shift systems, the European Working Time Directive and looser team structures. Of course, working with different people and seeing different ways of doing things can be educational, particularly with more senior trainees. However, if placements are too short, both teachers and learners have less time and incentive to invest in developing effective relationships. Learners may spend a disproportionate amount of time familiarising themselves with new colleagues and systems, leaving little time to consolidate learning.

Thinking point

Do your trainees have reasonable continuity with
(a) senior staff,
(b) patients?
If not, how might this be increased?

Discussion

(a) The introduction of named clinical and educational supervisors was designed to help provide continuity. Trainees may also find, or be given, mentors who can remain constant over a number of years. Some teams have managed to develop timetables which improve continuity. If you are in an educational leadership role, this may be something to consider.
(b) Trainees can be given projects to follow up individual patients during and after their treatment, which could be written up or presented to colleagues. Relationships can be developed with community colleagues so that learners see patients at different stages of their journey.

The Royal College of Physicians recommends that hospitals should organise rotas to encourage consistent team membership and that junior doctors should have a minimum of 6-month attachments to departments/specialties during training rotations [13].

Teaching and learning resources

Learning can be enhanced by the availability of appropriate teaching and learning resources (Table 1.4).

Thinking point

What learning resources are available for you and your students/trainees? How could they be enhanced?

Discussion

Sometimes grants are available from medical schools or other local sources to improve teaching resources.

The teaching climate

Having considered factors promoting learning, it is also worth considering what facilitates good teaching. The following are some factors that doctors on teaching courses have reported as helpful:

Good leadership
- Leaders who are knowledgeable and enthusiastic about teaching.
- An atmosphere of mutual respect and support.
- Clarity about the roles of different staff in teaching.
- A regular forum in which teachers can discuss teaching and the progress of individual trainees.

Table 1.4 Teaching and learning resources.

• Handbooks for students and trainees on placements	• Equipment modified for teaching, for example, double-headed stethoscope, slit lamp with extra eye piece
• Relevant books and journals	
• Posters	• Clinical images, video clips, protocols, book extracts stored on your mobile phone for use in teaching
• Models	
• Slide sets	
• Mannequins for skills practice	• Vodcasts and podcasts giving advice or teaching on core subjects
• Intranet page with local information, plus links to useful websites and e-learning modules	• Information about local training opportunities

Effective links
- With the medical school, Royal College and Foundation School.
- Regular updates, for example, information on changes to curricula or assessments.

Structural support
- Teaching and supervisory responsibilities recognised in job plans.
- Investment in teaching administration, facilities and resources.
- Training opportunities, study leave and funding.
- Recognition and reward for teaching.

Common difficulties cited by teachers include lack of time and conflicting demands.

What makes a good clinical teacher?

A meta-review of teaching strategies which have the most influence on learning concluded that three of the most important are
- setting relevant, specific and challenging goals;
- providing regular feedback;
- innovation – a deliberate and systematic attempt to improve the quality of learning [14].

Examples of the type of goals that can be set during clinical teaching are given in Chapter 2, and feedback is addressed in Chapter 3.

These and other characteristics of good clinical teachers are shown in Table 1.5 [15,16]. You may like to rate yourself against them and identify goals for improvement (which could already be areas of strength).

Table 1.5 Characteristics of effective clinical teachers.

Characteristic	Area of strength	Would like to develop
Demonstrate clinical competence		
Have a passion/enthusiasm for teaching		
Explain things clearly		
Are supportive to juniors		
Target teaching to the level of the learner(s)		
Provide specific, challenging tasks and goals		
Give regular feedback		
Show respect and compassion for learners		
Are accessible		
Use a broad repertoire of teaching methods		
Evaluate/reflect on teaching		

Thinking Point

What aspects of teaching do you enjoy most?
What rewards do you gain from teaching?
What kind of teacher would you like to be?

Discussion

Teachers often gain satisfaction from seeing learners improve, particularly if they work with them over a period of time. Teaching also stimulates the teacher's own learning and thus improves his or her knowledge and the standard of clinical care he or she provides.

In considering the kind of teacher you would like to be, you may have thought about your own teaching role models – those whom you would like to emulate.

This section has described how the way in which students and trainees are inducted into and supervised during a placement impacts on their motivation and learning. Setting an environment conducive to learning involves demonstrating enthusiasm for teaching, a team ethos, and supervision tailored to the individual's needs and stage of training. Learners also need a timetable that will provide appropriate opportunities for development. The immediate clinical supervisor can enhance the learning of students and trainees, and provides an important role model.

The following sections consider the input of patients and non-medical staff and outline some general principles and strategies for clinical teaching.

Be a yardstick of quality. Some people are not used to an environment where excellence is expected.

Steve Jobs, co-founder and chief executive of Apple

Involving patients in teaching

Patients are central to clinical teaching, and most studies show that they are willing to take part in teaching and perceive inherent benefits. For example, one study showed that patients felt more cared for, more comfortable and less anxious or bored when students were present. They felt better informed because of the discussion between doctor and student and were pleased to help future generations [17].

Often patients are relatively passive in the teaching process, but learners may benefit if they sometimes take a more active role.

Thinking point

Look at some of the roles which patients may play in clinical teaching (Table 1.6), and consider which ones(s) reflect your own approach.

Table 1.6 Patients' roles in teaching.

Patient role	Description
Clinical material	To be observed, examined and questioned
Problem	To be diagnosed and ultimately 'solved', with students learning from the process
Teacher	Asked to educate students about their experience and helping to shape what they learn
Assessor	Asked to give feedback to students
Resource	With a plethora of experience for students to draw on
Partner	Patient and doctor/student sharing their expertise about the condition.

Discussion

There is no single correct approach: different options may suit different clinical contexts and teaching purposes. However, you may like to consider incorporating additional roles to those that you already use. What would you aspire to? How practically might you achieve this? What would be your concerns?

Teachers may have concerns about lack of time and privacy, about patients being alarmed or confused by medical terminology, or learners losing face in front of the patient.

Examples of ways to involve patients actively include the following.

- Asking some to say a little more than strictly necessary, for example, about their experience of health care or how illness has affected their life.
- Asking the student to present the history in front of the patient and have the patient correct or add information.
- Asking patients to comment on non-medical aspects of the student's performance, for example, professionalism or communication skills.
- Identifying suitable patients and seeking their consent for extra roles, such as being a case study for a student project.

Another option is to encourage students and trainees to attend related activities (if acceptable to the group), for example,

- patient support groups;
- service user groups;

- patien education groups;
- parents' groups;
- carers' groups;
- service development meetings in which patients are involved.

In some specialties, it may be possible to arrange visits to patients at home, where learners can gain greater insight into their lives.

General principles
- Encourage direct contact between learners and patients.
- Keep the number of students low: split the group if necessary.
- Look out for non-verbal cues that patients are reluctant to engage with teaching even if they say yes.
- Ask learners questions which encourage them to explore and appreciate the impact of illness on the patient's life:
  - *What was the patient's main concern?*
  - *How has the patient's family been affected?*
- Be aware of patient fatigue.

'Everybody's a teacher if you listen.'

Doris Roberts, actress

Teacher comment

I learn a lot from parent groups where parents talk about how to deal with a 24-year old with severe autism. It gives me ideas that I can share with other parents.

Involving other disciplines in teaching

It is often useful to involve other disciplines (other medical specialties, health care professionals or biomedical scientists) in clinical teaching and learning. When doing so, you may wish to consider the following questions:
- What is the purpose? Are you looking for students to learn
  - specific skills;
  - about the colleague's roles;
  - about the patient's experience?

Everyone involved needs to be clear about the purpose and value of the experience.

- Is it feasible? Do your colleagues have the time, experience and skills to make it work?
- Are they willing? Or might they be willing with the right support? Be aware of the hierarchy (especially in hospitals) and the impact this may have on colleagues' willingness to teach. Some non-medical staff overestimate medical students'/trainees' knowledge and may need convincing of what they can offer.
- What information do they need? At a minimum, they will need to understand what they are expected to teach, how this fits into the curriculum and the learners' existing level of knowledge and competence.
- Can students/trainees from different disciplines learn together? There may be some skills which both groups require that could be learnt together.
- Can you reciprocate? Colleagues may have students of their own who need placements or teaching.

Learning/teaching opportunities
Consider what opportunities for mutual learning/teaching occur naturally, for example:
- with nurses, pharmacists or midwives on the wards;
- during case conferences or multi-agency meetings;
- during joint assessments of a patient.

The way in which you work with colleagues provides a model of inter-professional working. You may facilitate mutual learning, for example, by inviting them to give their perspective or specialised knowledge at appropriate points on a ward round. In addition, learners could be encouraged to
- follow a patient to referrals, seeing what others do and gaining insight into the patient's experience;
- shadow a non-medical colleague for a set period of time;
- talk to someone from another discipline about his or her training and role.

Colleagues from different professions and disciplines often have their own weekly or monthly teaching sessions. In some specialties, it may be appropriate to discuss opening (some of) their sessions to your learners and vice versa.

Teacher comment

I have my registrar and a senior pharmacist buddying up, so that they do joint assessments – sometimes a pharmacy assessment and sometimes a psychiatric assessment. They learn from each other's perspectives and they also teach junior medical staff together, and so model a multi-disciplinary team working approach.

Some principles of effective clinical teaching

- Give learners a genuine role in patient care, wherever possible. Responsibility is a great motivator.
- Where this is not possible, engage them actively in meaningful tasks and add value by reviewing their learning.
- Aim to gradually increase the learners' level of responsibility and autonomy, offering gradually diminishing levels of support as they gain in confidence and competence.
- Help learners to see the wood for the trees. Whilst the details of individual cases are important, learners also need to see the overall picture. Help them to look for patterns and trends and to understand the overall aims of investigation and management.
- Focus on the development of clinical thinking rather than factual recall. So, for example, ask *'What in this patient would lead you to be concerned about heart disease?'* rather than *'Tell me the five most common causes of heart disease'*.

'The mediocre teacher tells. The good teacher explains. The superior teacher demonstrates. The great teacher inspires.'

William Arthur Ward, writer

Useful strategies for clinical teaching

- **Explicate practice:** Explain what you are doing and why.
- **Prompt observation:** Help learners to notice more about the patient or your practice.
- **Make comparisons:** Draw attention to similarities and differences in the presentation, investigation and management of patients. *This helps learners to understand the variation within and between different pathologies and how care is tailored to the individual.*
- **Stimulate thinking:** Ask learners to make sense of what they see/hear. Invite them to form differential diagnoses or management plans rather than just describing signs and symptoms.
- **Draw out general principles** from specific patients.
- **Link theory and practice:** Draw on learners' existing theoretical knowledge and help them make links to the patients they see.
- **Share the tricks of the trade:** Tell learners the mnemonics you use, lessons you learnt the hard way or patient anecdotes that convey an important message.

- **Signpost**: Alert learners to colleagues, services or resources that they can access to further their learning.
- **Listen for cues**: Often trainees will reveal their concerns and difficulties in throw away comments that can easily be missed.

Comments from Teachers *and Learners*

I always treat the registrars as potential consultant colleagues.

I tell students what I expect them to be able to do at 1 week, 4 weeks, 2 months, etc. and also get them to comment on whether that feels reasonable and make it clear that they may go faster or slower and that we will keep things under review.

We have kept our firm structure – we have had to fight for it but we still work with our juniors regularly.

Some people leave medical school with inadequate knowledge and fail to grasp the concept that they are now doctors and not students. They are paid to provide a service to patients and should strive to develop themselves without expecting everything to be 'taught'.

I tell people at the start that there are no wrong answers.

Students are invited to the Echo meeting, but it took us a long time to realise that they did not understand hardly anything that was going on and we did not make any attempt to include them or to explain things to them.

We cancel the ENT clinics in the first week of a new rotation, so that we can teach the juniors the skills they need before starting.

Every firm could think about what sorts of tasks medical students could do that would be useful to them.

Most people are good teachers if you ask them to teach something specific: you need to work out what you want.

I was asked to do something that I am not qualified to do. Some consultants have strong personalities and it can be quite hard to resist sometimes.

I appreciated my consultant checking in with me every day to see how I was getting on.

I was shouted at a lot as a junior. You immediately panic and do not want to be involved with that person anymore – I lost a lot of confidence.

The registrars almost become like a mentor to you and are often in the best position to assess your progression.

The best supervisors are skilled in drawing out ideas, aspirations and stumbling blocks and creative in bringing about alternative regimes, pathways and attitudes.

Five tips for clinical teaching which do not take time or money

- **Show your enthusiasm**: A passion for your work and teaching will infect others.
- **Excel at your job**: You are role model, so set a standard of practice to which you would be happy for your learners to aspire.
- **Have high (but realistic) expectations**: People usually live up to them.
- **Exploit every opportunity**: Much useful learning can take place whilst walking from one ward to the next, when a patient cancels or over a coffee.
- **Treat everyone as part of the team**: Involving students and trainees in the life of the team builds rapport and commitment even in short placements.

References

[1] Eraut M, Alderton J, Cole G, Senker P. Development of Knowledge and Skills in Employment: Research Report No. 5. University of Sussex Institute of Education; 1998.

[2] Hattie J. Teachers make a difference. What is the research evidence? Presentation to the Australian Council for Educational Research; 2003. www.acer.edu.au /documents/RC2003_Hattie_TeachersMakeADifference.pdf [accessed on 19 July 2013].

[3] King S, David M. *Training within the organization: a study of company policy and procedures for the systematic training of operators and supervisors.* London: Tavistock Publishers; 1964. p 126.

[4] Lempp H, Seale C. The hidden curriculum in undergraduate medical education: qualitative study of medical students' perceptions of teaching. *BMJ* 2004; 329:770.

[5] Lempp H, Cochrane M, Rees J. A qualitative study of the perceptions and experiences of pre-registration house officers on teamwork and support. *BMC Med Educ* 2005; 5:10.

[6] Seabrook M. Apprenticeship or university education? A study of change in one medical school. Unpublished PhD thesis. University of London; 2002.

[7] Seabrook MA. Intimidation in medical education: students' and teachers' perspectives. *Stud High Educ* 2004; 29:59–74.

[8] Rotem A, Godwin P, Du J. Learning in hospital settings. *Teach Learn Med* 1995; 7(4):211–217.

[9] Williams DJP. Medication Errors. *J R Coll Physicians Edinb* 2007; 37:343–346

[10] Sexton JB, Thomas EJ, Helmreich RL. Error, stress, and teamwork in medicine and aviation: cross sectional surveys. *BMJ* 2000; 320(7237):745–749.

[11] For a summary of evidence, see Miller R. *Greater Expectations to improve student learning (briefing paper).* Washington, DC: Association of American Colleges and Universities; 2001.

[12] Hyland T, Johnson S. Of cabbages and key skills: exploding the mythology of core transferable skills in post-school education. *J Further High Educ* 1998; 22(2): 163–172.

[13] Royal College of Physicians. RCP briefing. Health reforms: education, training and workforce issues. September 2011.

[14] Hattie J. Influences on Student Learning. Inaugural Professorial Lecture. University of Auckland; 1999. www.education.auckland.ac.nz/uoa/home/about /staff/j.hattie/hattie-papers-download/influences [accessed on 19 July 2013].

[15] Ramsden P. *Learning to teach in higher education*. Routledge: New York; 2003.

[16] Irby DM, Papadakis M. Does good clinical teaching really make a difference? *Am J Med* 2001; 110:231–232.

[17] Ashley P, Rhodes N, Sari-Kouzel H, Mukherjee A, Dornan T. 'They've all got to learn'. Medical students' learning from patients in ambulatory (outpatient and general practice) consultations. *Med Teach* 2009; 31(2):e24–e31.

Chapter 2 **Teaching in clinical contexts**

Teaching on ward rounds

Some doctors distinguish between business and teaching ward rounds. In reality, they are probably two ends of a spectrum with all rounds including elements of business and learning (if not explicit teaching) in varying proportions. In this book, there is a separate chapter on bedside teaching where the main purpose is teaching and the teacher and learners may not have service responsibility for the patients involved. In this chapter, the focus is on how learning can be incorporated into routine ward rounds.

General principles
- Establish an atmosphere in which you set high standards of care and support and encourage trainees to achieve them.
- Be aware of maintaining the credibility of trainees and students in the eyes of the patient: patients want to have confidence in those who are looking after them.
- Aim for learners to understand, not just know, what is being done for the patient. It will make the experience meaningful for them and should result in better care for your patients.
- Consider how much to discuss at the bedside and what is better discussed before/after/away from the bed. Avoid talking across the patient or discussing unrelated issues in front of them.
- Clarify roles: assign or negotiate who will present each patient, take notes, lead the consultation, etc. Vary these roles appropriately so that everyone gets opportunities and experience relevant to their level of training.

How to Teach in Clinical Settings, First Edition. Mary Seabrook.
© 2014 John Wiley & Sons, Ltd. Published 2014 by John Wiley & Sons, Ltd.

'I desire no other epitaph. . . than the statement that I taught medical students in the wards, as I regard this as by far the most useful and important work I have been called upon to do.'

Sir William Osler, Professor of Medicine

Comments from Teachers *and Learners*

When I first started as a consultant, I found the ward rounds very pressurised. Then, I decided that I was going to take the time I needed for every patient. Now, I feel more in control and I am sure that the time I invest is saved in other ways.

I think that students can learn a lot by osmosis, but perhaps I ought to find out from them what they have learnt and get them more involved in interviewing patients.

I find that explaining things to students and junior doctors also helps me to think through the patient's problems and plan.

To give the juniors more ownership, I get the SHO to be in the hot seat for the first half of the ward round. She presents the patients and writes in the notes, while the F2 acts as a runner. Then, they swap over for the second half.

I find that it takes several weeks for students on the ward round to start to ask questions and believe that you are not going to show them up.

On ward rounds, I try to discuss a similar theme with each patient, for example, the character of the pulse, heart sounds or ECGs [electrocardiograms]. This repetition improves the retention of the learning topic.

I think that ward rounds can be very helpful in mentoring all sorts of generic skills such as communication, teamwork, respect and compassion. Interprofessional learning can often be accomplished using the whole of the multi-disciplinary team.

As a student, everyone tries to avoid standing to the right of the patient because you know that if you stand there, you will get picked on to examine in front of everyone!

If people set you homework, they do need to tell you when they are going to check on it, otherwise, although I intend to do it, I don't.

What is really useful is when you have a consultant-supervised rather than a consultant-led ward round, and you get to lead on patients.

As a first-year registrar, the trouble with being critiqued quite heavily in front of juniors is that it starts to undermine their faith in your decisions. I spoke to the consultant about it.

Useful strategies

The following is a list of strategies, many of which you may already use, and others you might wish to incorporate (as time allows), to enhance the educational value of ward rounds.

Planning

- Consider asking senior trainees to decide the order of the round to help them develop their prioritisation and organisational skills.
- Pick a focus for the ward round or a topic of the week, for example,
  - examination of the abdomen;
  - interpretation of blood results;
  - pharmaceutical management.
- Give yourself a teaching goal, for example, to give everyone the opportunity to listen to a chest/interpret an X-ray.
- Allocate certain patients as 'teaching cases' where you will spend slightly longer.
- Check knowledge/experience before starting (especially if you do not know the learners) and as you go round:
  - *'Have you had any previous experience in vascular medicine?'*
  - *'Has anyone been involved in Do Not Resuscitate decisions?'*

Giving roles

- Ask each trainee to present at least one patient. This could increase week by week as he or she progresses.
- Ask each trainee to lead a consultation and suggest a management plan. As a team, discuss and agree immediate management and get the same person to conclude the consultation.
- Have senior speciality trainees (STs) lead the ward round (or part thereof), with you available for consultation: this is good preparation for consultant responsibilities. Afterwards, meet with the STs privately to review their management of the team.

Developing observational skills

- Have students/trainees make observations from the foot of the bed before approaching the patient.
- Give a question to focus their observations/review, for example,
  - *'So, what are we looking for in a patient who has just had a major operation?'*
  - *'When examining a patient with lower abdominal pain, what are we thinking of?'*

- Have them evaluate the overall trend in the patients' observations/investigations: *'what do the observations tell us at a glance?'*

Prompting thinking
- Probe understanding:
  - *'Why do you think that her oedema has got worse?'*
  - *'Do you know why warfarin might have been withheld?'*
- Help them to see the bigger picture:
  - *'What is the main issue here?'*
  - *'What kind of clinical picture is this?'*
- Ask members of the team to explain things to more junior members (e.g. FY1 to fifth-year student, ST4 to FY2): *this involves all levels appropriately and will often happen spontaneously.*
- Occasionally, ask *'What have you learnt from this patient?'* This encourages students/trainees to make their learning explicit and also gives you feedback on their understanding.

Explaining and demonstrating
- Encourage learners to observe you with the patient. *Sometimes, they are so busy taking or reviewing the patient's notes that they miss opportunities to learn from observing you and the patient.*
- Demonstrate a team approach by involving other disciplines appropriately in the round.
- Explain your thinking:
  - *'I am going to increase his dose to 100 mg because . . . '*
- Be open about your dilemmas:
  - *'The difficulty here is trying to balance medication against quality of life.'*
- Identify patterns which help learners make sense of what they see:
  - *'So we have three examples of different complications of hernia today . . . two common and one much rarer. . . '*
  - *'Mrs X is a classic case of clinical depression, whereas Mr B also has psychotic symptoms.'*

Setting learning tasks
- Students may be better seeing only a few patients and then being given learning tasks, ideally ones that contribute to patient care as well:
  - *'Call the GP to get background information.'*
  - *'We saw that this patient has anaemia – go and find out about the potential causes, and come and join us again when you are ready.'*

- Set challenges during or after the ward round:
  - *'Let's look up side effects and drug interactions of phenytoin.'*
  - *'Come back later and see if you can feel the patient's spleen.'*

Other options
- Periodically review the patient's notes immediately after seeing the patient and give feedback.
- Pause at times during the round to allow time for questions to emerge naturally. This may seem difficult given the pressure of work, but waiting even a few seconds can open up opportunities for learning.
- Have a 'working coffee' half way round (or at the end). This allows informal discussion of cases and an opportunity for questions. It promotes a team ethos, helps trainees to consolidate information and gives renewed energy for the rest of the round/jobs.
- At the end of the round, get trainees to discuss how they will prioritise their tasks, reviewing which are most urgent. *Prioritisation is often omitted from teaching but can be one of the most difficult aspects for trainees to learn.*

I like a teacher who gives you something to take home to think about besides homework.

Lily Tomlin, actress and comedian

What you teach unwittingly
Studies have shown that students gradually acquire professional values during the apprenticeship element of their training.[1] What is learnt, usually unconsciously, through this process of professional socialisation is sometimes termed the *hidden curriculum*. Whilst it is a subtle and complex process, the model set by the teacher is highly influential. Students and trainees learn what is acceptable by seeing the example of their seniors (Box 2.1). In fact, the General Medical Council goes so far as to say that

> The example of the teacher is the most powerful influence upon the standards of conduct and practice of every trainee [1].

Therefore, it is worth reflecting on the values that you may transmit to learners.

---

[1] There is a substantial literature on professional socialization in medicine, from classic studies by Merton (1957) and Becker (1961) to more recent contributions from Hafferty (1991) and Sinclair (1997).

Box 2.1 The hidden curriculum

During an elderly care ward round, the consultant came across a patient who was having difficulty hearing. He found her hearing aid and saw that it was damaged. He challenged two of the students to try to mend it and waited until it was working again before talking to the patient.

The consultant demonstrated the importance he attached to communicating with the patient by taking time to make this possible, and in doing so engaged the trainees in solving a practical problem.

Thinking point

Consider the questions in Table 2.1 – the answers may reveal something about the values inherent in your practice. Warning! – the espoused values of individuals (what they say is important) and the values evident in their practice (what they actually do) are often different [2].

Table 2.1 Values in practice.

- Do you allow time for questions from the patient?
- Do you seek opinions from non-medical staff?
- Do you see patients even if there is nothing medical to be done for them?
- Do you avoid noticing patients trying to get your attention?
- Do you give false reassurance?
- Do you explain mistakes which have been made to the patient?
- Do you continue the ward round over an empty bed if the patient is absent?
- Do you avoid meeting relatives?
- Do you credit colleagues when they have made a difference?

Discussion

If any of the questions made you feel angry or defensive, it may be because you do not agree with the implicit values behind the questions. (Values vary between specialities – if, as a student, you sometimes felt that you did not fit into a certain speciality, it may have been due to a clash of values).

Alternatively, these may be the areas where there is some mismatch between your espoused (ideal) values and current practice – perhaps because of the pressures of the job.

When doctors are asked about the people who inspired them, they often talk, not so much about their skills or knowledge, but about the kind of people they were.

Thinking point

Think of one or more colleagues whom you particularly respected during your own training. What were the qualities you admired?

Discussion

You may like to consider how you do, or could, incorporate those qualities into your own practice.

The psychiatric ward round

Psychiatric ward rounds often come as a surprise to students who are used to hospital-style ward rounds. You may need to brief them on the format or allow them to observe a round before getting actively involved.

Before the ward round

Discuss the trainees'/students' role, clarifying or negotiating whether they are there as observers or participants. If observers, consider what they could focus on; if participants, discuss how they will contribute, for example, by presenting patients or chairing all or part of the meeting (Box 2.2).

During the ward round

There are distinct phases of the ward round: before the patient arrives, whilst the patient and accompanying person(s) are present and after they have left.

Box 2.2 A simple solution

Dr Rashid suggested that her Registrar lead the ward round. He was keen to do this to gain experience before applying for consultant posts. However, after handing over the chair, Dr Rashid found that the team still looked to her for leadership. A colleague suggested that she move seats from that adjacent to the Registrar to one on the other side of the group. She tried this and found that it solved the problem.

Depending on their level, roles for trainees or students might include the following:

1. Before the patient's arrival
   - Identifying the different types of information brought to the meeting by each discipline
   - Presenting, or giving information or opinions about, patients
   - Identifying what needs to be elicited from/ discussed with/ communicated to the patient.

2. When the patient is present
   You may want to focus the learners' attention by suggesting
   - specific things to observe and note about the patient's appearance or behaviour;
   - signs and symptoms to look out for relevant to current teaching;
   - a role in the patient's record keeping;
   - a role in the discussion with the patient, which may be consistent across all patients, or vary with each patient;
   - noticing how each consultation is managed, including specific questions asked and language used.

3. After the patient has left
   You could summarise key issues or learning points or elicit these from the learner(s). Consider also using some of the strategies listed under the section on Handover meetings.

After the meeting

It is helpful to allow a few minutes for the student/trainee to debrief. Invite him or her to comment on the round, review his or her role and ask questions. It may be interesting to discuss how this round compares to others he or she has seen previously and to reflect on how decisions were made.

Handover meetings, board rounds and bench rounds

During these meetings, each patient is reviewed, usually briefly. The educational value can be increased by strategies such as the following:

- Encourage analysis of case presentations by asking the team:
  - '*What would you include in the differential diagnosis?*'
  - '*What should we do next?*'
- Draw general principles from specific cases:
  - '*Whenever you see a patient like this, remember your Sepsis Six.*'
  - '*What is the first line therapy for COPD?*'

- Change the goalposts:
  - ○ *'What would you do if the patient was pregnant/80 years old/male/had diabetes?'*

  This helps trainees to understand how management is tailored to the patient.
- Ask for evidence:
  - ○ *'How do you know it is a pulmonary embolism?'*
  - ○ *'What abnormalities are present within the epidermis which suggest skin failure?'*
- Encourage application of knowledge:
  - ○ *'What yeast is it most likely to be?'*
  - ○ *'Why is she at high risk for endometrial cancer? What is the mechanism?'*
- Identify the key issue:
  - ○ *'Do we need to admit her or can we let her go home?'*
  - ○ Or, ask *'What is the key issue here?'*
- Seek and compare opinions on the best approach by asking:
  - ○ More than one consultant (if available): *the team learn that there are different views and may not be one right answer.*
  - ○ Other professionals: *this helps trainees and students to understand their roles and contribution to care.*
  - ○ Trainees: *This encourages learners to pay attention to every case.*
  - ○ Students: *sometimes appropriate, but may be time-consuming and stressful for them. You may prefer one of your team to discuss key issues with them afterwards.*
  - ○ Everyone: take a vote:
    - *'Who would section her?'*
    - *'Who thinks she needs a CT scan?'*

  Ask someone on each side for their reasoning.
- Share your experience, for example, describe similar cases you have seen, how you would approach a particular problem, or how similar cases would be managed in India/Australia/Egypt.
- During the meeting, note any issues or patients who might provide good teaching opportunities later.

After the meeting, you could:
- give an overview or comment on specific themes:
  - ○ *'So we have got the whole spectrum of abruption in one day.'*
- clarify patients needing senior review and who will review each.
- take 5–10 minutes to review a topic relevant to one of the patients with selected trainees or students.
- select relevant trainees to see a patient with you.
- signpost learning opportunities, such as good patients to clerk, relevant reading.

Comments from Teachers *and Learners*

The different grades of doctors hand over very differently – juniors hand over tasks, trainees hand over patients and consultants hand over problems – and you have to try to combine these all together.

I found the board rounds in geriatrics very useful because we went through each patient's discharge and heard from the occupational therapists, doctors and nurses and I understood their role much better.

Bedside teaching

Bedside teaching, when not part of a ward round, is usually to enable students/ trainees to learn specific clinical skills, or as examination practice. Formal teaching sessions may also sometimes be used for bedside teaching (Box 2.3).

Preparation

- To determine the focus and level of the teaching, you may wish to
  - check out the learners' agenda: what do they want to learn/practise?
  - check their previous experience;
  - consider what you think they need most (perhaps from observing them clinically);
  - consult their curriculum;
  - review the available patients (see below).
- Clarify your objectives. Are you going to focus on some or all of
  - the elicitation of signs and/or symptoms?
  - the presentation of findings?
  - the interpretation and meaning of the findings?
  - the quality of the differential diagnosis?
  - plans for further investigation and management?
- If you have weekly teaching, then plan a series of topics, preferably in consultation with the learners. You may need some flexibility to adapt to the available patients.
- Encourage the learners to come prepared:
  - '*Next week we will be focusing on neurological examination, so make sure you know your peripheral nerve pathways before then.*'
  - If you are teaching an examination technique which is new to students, you may want to hold a formal teaching session first in which they can practise on each other or on mannequins.

Box 2.3 An unplanned session

Dr Petrovich, an associate specialist working in Ear, Nose & Throat, had prepared a PowerPoint presentation for a teaching session for the juniors. In the event, only one ST3 and one ST4 arrived. He changed his plans and asked them each to go and clerk a patient and return in 15 minutes. He then accompanied them to the bedside where they presented their findings. He invited the patients to add or correct information or ask questions. He checked some of the findings directly and then discussed the doctors' management plans, asking them to justify their decisions. Feedback from the doctors was that this was a particularly useful session.

- Consider whether you want to see learners clerking the patient, or just to hear their presentations.
- Plan what will take place at the patient's bedside and what away from the patient. You may need to identify/book a nearby room.

Aspects to consider when selecting patients
- how ill they are and how much they can cope with;
- if in hospital, how long they are likely to be there (and how much follow up you want);
- their relevance to your learners: for example, when teaching students, you may want patients with typical presentations of common conditions; whereas, for STs, you might prefer atypical presentations or rarer conditions;
- their personality and characteristics (Box 2.4): again, depending on the level of the trainee. You might encourage new students by allocating them the more straightforward patients whilst challenging senior trainees with patients who are deaf or have a learning disability.

Briefing patients
- Seek consent from patients before the teaching, explaining how you will conduct the teaching and how long it will take.
- Let them know if you do not want them to disclose their diagnosis.
- Advise them that not everything that is discussed will be applicable to them and that you will give them an opportunity for questions afterwards.
- Consider whether they might have an active role in feedback (see below).

Structure for bedside teaching
Often it is useful to think in terms of a simple three-part structure:
1. the briefing (preparing the learner);
2. at the bedside (the practical experience);
3. the de-briefing (consolidating and extending the learning).
The following sections contain suggestions as to what you might want to include at each stage.

Box 2.4 Choosing the 'right' patient

A surgeon had organised bedside teaching on the subject of breast examination for a group of four final year students. They approached the bed where the patient whom he had briefed was waiting with her husband. Asking her to undo her top, she did so, immediately diffusing the students' anxiety by telling them: 'I am afraid that my glamour modelling days are over!'

1. The briefing
   - explain the aims of the teaching and how you intend to conduct the session:
     - *'We are going to practise examining patients with chest conditions today, so I have four patients for you to see and I am going to ask one of you to lead on each.'*
   - explain what you expect of them
     - *'I want you to take a history and then present the key findings and your differential diagnosis.'*
     - *'I expect you to do a focused examination and present your findings succinctly.'* If they are taking an examination shortly, you can specify *'present your findings to the examiner'* – but beware of over-emphasising the assessment element unless your teaching is specifically examination practice (see p. 36). It can add unnecessary pressure and give an implicit message that learning is primarily to pass examinations rather than for their own development or to improve patient care.
   - recap relevant theoretical knowledge (Box 2.5):
     - *'What are the red flag symptoms that you will be looking for?'*
     - *'What risk factors will you check?'*
   - rehearse what they will do:
     - *'So, before we start, let's recap the main stages of the upper limb examination.'*
   - establish what constitutes good practice:
     - *'So, what are the dos and don'ts of taking a sexual history?'*
     - *'What makes a mini-mental state examination effective?'*

Box 2.5 Briefing before bedside teaching

Dr Chopra, an ST4 in ophthalmology, checked the group's experience of visual field examination, and realising that it was limited, decided to do a quick review. She drew a pair of eyes and asked the group for the next part of the anatomical pathway to the brain. As they made suggestions, she added the features and names to the diagram. Then, she asked 'If you had a lesion in one of these areas, where in the visual field would the defect be?' She asked the group to work in pairs on this and then after a couple of minutes, went through their answers, drawing up the visual fields affected, and telling them common causes of each defect (see Figure 2.1, original was in three colours).

2. At the bedside
   - Depending on the aims of your teaching, you may either:
     - go round together, getting learners to clerk and present patients in front of you;
     - ask them to see the patients independently/in pairs, then go round together, getting them to present their findings for review.

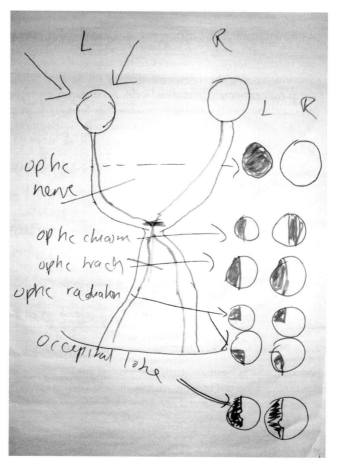

Figure 2.1 Flipchart from briefing session.

- Structure your session so that everyone is involved in both the practical activities and your questioning.
- You could divide up the hands-on learning into small sections and rotate regularly to keep everyone involved and make it less daunting for individuals.
- Consider how to involve the learners who are not examining or taking a history, for example,
  - asking them questions;
  - asking them to give feedback on their peers' technique.
- Aim to be constructive and encouraging so that learners feel comfortable enough to ask questions and make mistakes. The only exception to this is if you are aiming to simulate examination conditions (see p. 36).
- Give tips that you have found useful, for example, memory aids or structures for history taking or examination (Box 2.6).

3. De-briefing
   This is an opportunity to review the learning and plan further development:
   - Ask an open question to elicit learners' immediate thoughts or concerns:
     - 'How was that?'
   - Invite questions.
   - Explain any points that were not fully explained at the bedside.
   - Ask the trainees what they have gained from the session.
   - Give feedback – if this has not been done already.
   - Recap on the main learning points.
   - Ask for comments on the way the teaching was conducted.

Box 2.6 Drawing on personal experience

An FY2 on a paediatric rotation had two students who wanted to prepare for their Objective Structured Clinical Examinations. He enlisted the help of a 14-year-old girl with cystic fibrosis and asked the students to take a history, then return and present their findings. He gave feedback on their presentations, and suggested a structure that he found helpful. He asked each in turn to examine the respiratory system, giving a running commentary as to what they were looking for, and summarising their findings at the end. They then left the bedside, and the FY2 critiqued their examination skills. He described his own experience during finals and gave tips on OSCE technique and preparation.

- Discuss what topics learners need to know more about.
- Discuss further skills they would like to acquire/practise.
- Recommend useful sources of information and discuss opportunities for further practical experience.
- Suggest a target:
  - *'I would like you each to examine three more patients with chest conditions this week.'*
- Ask about priorities for future teaching.

Feedback at the bedside

- Consider when to give feedback. This may depend on the level of the trainee: you may want to wait until the end and then comment on the overall sequence and structure of the examination or you might prefer to intervene to correct or improve technique as they proceed.
- Endeavour to give feedback sensitively – both patients and learners can be embarrassed by inappropriate or overly critical feedback.
- It may be more effective to prioritise a few important points rather than correcting everything.
- Some feedback can be done subtly, for example, by asking several people in the group to demonstrate and then highlighting aspects of good practice from each (Box 2.7).

Box 2.7 Feedback at the bedside

Dr Yin, a medical ST5, arranged an hour's bedside teaching with four final year students approaching their final examinations. She had asked them which examinations they wished to practise: two chose neurological, one cardiac and one abdominal.

She selected four relevant patients, and the group went round, with the relevant student examining and taking a focused history within a given time limit. When time was up, they were asked to summarise their findings. The other students were asked to critique the examination technique. Dr Yin gave guidance as to technique and asked questions focusing on the interpretation of the examination findings. She also gave her own summary of the findings which acted as a model for the students to emulate. Questions about the specific patient were addressed to the lead student, more general questions about the condition to those observing.

At the end of the session, Dr Yin asked each student what they had learnt and what they would do next to improve.

Peer Feedback

A fairly common method is to ask learners to critique each other.

Thinking point

From your experience, what are the advantages and disadvantages of this method? How could its effectiveness be improved?

Discussion

On the positive side, it gives everyone a role throughout the session. It focuses their attention, and they can also learn how to give feedback. On the other hand, they may not know enough to critique accurately or they may be reluctant to give honest feedback to peers.

To make the process effective, you might consider
- moving away from the patient for the feedback: you can always return if necessary;
- asking observers to define what they will be looking for (before starting);
- allocating roles: for example, one person to be the 'dove' – commenting on what was done well, another the 'hawk' – noting improvements needed;
- getting learners to act as examiners: giving them the marking form to complete whilst their colleague is examining;
- providing a structure, for example,
  - A to comment on the sequence of the examination/history taking,
  - B on the examination technique/nature of the questions,
  - C on instructions to and communication with the patient,
  - D to make one constructive suggestion for improvement.

You could give each student a card describing the criteria for good practice in his or her area to inform the feedback. When the next person examines, students could swap cards and comment on a different area.

The latter ideas are particularly helpful for novices as they help them to understand what constitutes good practice.

Patient Feedback

You could ask the patient to feed back to the learners. If so, discuss with the patient beforehand: some may be uncomfortable with the role, whilst others may welcome the opportunity or even have professional skills in this area. Clarify when and how they will feed back (e.g. to you or direct to the learner, on paper or in person).

They could comment on areas such as
- clarity of instructions;
- whether they felt listened to;
- clarity of explanation;
- comfort of the examination;
- accuracy of the trainee's summary;
- whether they felt able to ask questions and express concerns.

Modelling
You could demonstrate good practice, for example, giving your own summary of examination findings or showing learners your examination technique.

Repeat Performance
It is often useful to give the learner a chance to incorporate feedback immediately. So, after reviewing examination technique, get the learner to practise it again in the correct way (on the same or a different patient). Or, allow another attempt to summarise the findings succinctly. This will provide immediate reinforcement of the corrected or improved technique, and, hopefully, a sense of achievement for both of you.

A master can tell you what he expects of you. A teacher, though, awakens your own expectations.

Patricia Neal, actress

Examination practice at the bedside
One of the key differences between routine bedside teaching and preparing trainees for examinations is that in the latter, you may wish to play the role of the examiner. If this is the case, make it clear to both the trainee and patient that you are playing a role, so that they understand that the normal rules of engagement have changed. You can then be more formal and demanding during the observation. Afterwards, revert back to your normal self for the feedback.

Useful strategies
- Ask the trainee to specify what kind of examiner he or she would like you to enact. For example, he or she may like you to be kind and friendly, demanding or awkward. *Trainees will often know implicitly what stage they are at and what kind of practice will help them.*

- Get the trainees to act as examiners. *Observing peers from an examiner's perspective helps them to understand what examiners are looking for and what comes across well or badly.*
- Get trainees to use the real examination mark sheets, if available. If not, get them to generate their own. *This helps them to identify and recognise the criteria for good practice.*
- Give trainees a set time to present the patient and have one of the group time them on their mobile phone.
- If you have been an examiner recently, explain what you look for, giving examples of good or poor practice you have seen.

Learner quote

Students are not worried about practising history taking because you can practise that on your friends using the OSCE book. They want to practise examination techniques.

Teaching in clinics

The waiting room is full, the receptionists getting agitated. You have 20 patients to see and two students who you have never seen before have arrived for teaching. They are already looking bored, sat in the corner and not asking any questions. They are expecting another tedious afternoon observing multiple consultations, and wondering how soon they dare ask you to sign their log book before going home.

So, how can you make this a productive experience for the students and still see 20 patients without running too far over time? Learners' perceptions of what affects the effectiveness of teaching in Outpatients is given in Table 2.2.

General principles

- **Facilitate attendance**: Doctors often comment that trainees and students do not attend enough clinics: trainees may find it difficult to escape ward work, whilst students are sometimes deterred by past experiences of sitting passively through long clinics. Discuss with trainees how they can make time to attend.
- **Learners need not attend the entire clinic or see every patient**: Coming for an hour, or to clerk and present two patients, may be more manageable for trainees, more motivating for students and easier for you.
- **Establish need**: Take a few minutes at the start to explore the learners' experience and knowledge in order to establish how they would benefit most from the clinic.
- **Set goals**: Ask learners what they hope to gain from the clinic, and advise them if it is realistic. If learners are unclear of their goals – and they are often surprised by the question – give them a few minutes to think about

Table 2.2 Learners' perceptions of factors affecting the effectiveness of teaching in outpatients.

Availability and effectiveness of teachers
Time for teaching
Meaningful participation, not just observation
Students having their own patient caseload, with appropriate responsibility
  and supervision
Longitudinal attachments, providing continuity with patients

Data from Reference 3.

it, or suggest options. Having a specific goal will help the trainee/student to focus, but need not exclude other areas of interest that may arise.

- **Focus on what is best learnt in clinic**: For example, many doctors find clinics the best place to demonstrate clinical signs. It can also be a good place to teach examination technique, including intimate examinations.
- **Provide an active role**: learning is increased when individuals are actively involved, gaining hands on experience under supervision, or thinking about what they are seeing (Box 2.8).
- **Make resources available**: For example, a computer with Internet access, definitive texts, anatomical posters or models can support learning.
- **Involve others**: Learners could spend time with junior colleagues or other disciplines working in the clinic arena.

Remember: you may not always have time to teach but that does not mean that students are not learning. They can gain a lot from seeing how patients present and watching how you conduct the consultations (Box 2.9).

Box 2.8 Practical involvement

Mr Hammond, orthopaedic surgeon, had an F2, Sarah, in clinic. He summarised the first patient's notes and explained the management aim and the need to assess the patient's elbow (which he thought would be useful to her in A&E). He brought up the X-rays, highlighting the key features and asking, 'What would that make it?' Sarah suggested osteoarthritis. Mr Hammond agreed, elaborating a little and noting various points on the X-ray. They went to see the patient and he examined her elbow function and explained that she would need an injection.

In a separate room, Mr Hammond drew a diagram of the elbow joint and explained the surface anatomy, getting Sarah to feel on her own elbow. Returning to the patient, with her permission, he drew the surface anatomy which Sarah then felt, before giving the injection. Afterwards, he suggested that she listen into the letter he was dictating as it would give her a summary.

Box 2.9 Two for the price of one

A urology ST5 used a computer animation showing a nephrectomy to explain the procedure to her patient. She described the benefits and risks and answered questions from the patient, at the same time educating two students who were observing.

Thinking point

Imagine that you are a consultant with two third-year medical students and an ST5 in clinic. How would you organise the clinic and allocate patients?

Discussion

Of course, there is no right answer and it will depend partly on what space is available. Consider whether you would want to keep the students together or split them up. Would you involve your ST 5 in teaching? What would be the benefits and drawbacks? You might also want to refer the students' curriculum or ask them what they need to learn.

Clinics vary greatly in terms of the number of patients, length of appointments and space available: not all the suggestions in this chapter will be feasible for everyone, but hopefully, some can work for you. The first section considers supervision of trainees in parallel clinics and the second, one considers students or trainees who are supernumerary.

Supervising trainees in parallel clinics

- Consider the allocation of patients: you may want learners at a particular level to focus on different types of patients:
  - new versus follow ups;
  - complex versus routine;
  - common versus unusual diagnoses;
  - focused on a particular condition(s) or varied;
  - random allocation.

    Alternatively, ask trainees to look through the clinic list the day before and identify patients they would like to see. *This encourages preparation and greater ownership of their learning.*
- Pre-clinic review:
  - Look through the patients' notes before clinic and discuss consultation aims and strategies with the trainee.
  - Remind trainees of important information, for example, investigation, referral or discharge criteria.
- Clarify supervision arrangements:
  - Do you expect trainees to present every patient or just those for whom they would like advice or a second opinion?
  - Alternatively, you may specify certain criteria for patients you would like to review, for example, all new patients or all they intend to discharge.
- You can build in progression by allowing more independence or access to more complex patients as they gain in competence.

- Ask colleagues in the clinic to alert the trainees/students if they have any interesting or unusual patients.
- Ask trainees to take a student for a set length of time and teach them a specific skill: this will help the trainees too as teaching someone else is one of the best ways of learning yourself.
- If you have several trainees, you may find it effective to focus mainly (or even entirely) on supervision – dividing the patients between your trainees, having them present to you, reviewing their plans and seeing the patient yourself where necessary.
- Post-clinic review: Meet with trainees after the clinic to review each patient briefly or to debrief (Table 2.3). *This allows you to keep track of your patients and check that they have been appropriately managed, as well as identifying educational issues and resolving queries. Trainees who have experienced these meetings invariably rate them highly.*
- After the clinic, you can encourage trainees to notice similarities and differences between patients, for example, patients at different stages on a disease pathway or having different treatments for the same condition.

Effective questioning on presented cases
Avoid asking only for factual details about patients, and help learners to develop using some of the following strategies:

To hone analysis and presentation
- Ask questions to help learners evaluate and synthesise information. (Inexperienced students/trainees tend to present a lot of unsifted information and may need help to become more selective and analytical):
  - *'So, summarise the key positive and negative findings and your differential diagnosis.'*
  - *'How do the investigations results inform your management plan?'*
- Give further practice in summarising succinctly:
  - *'Now present the patient again in half the time.'*
  - *'Summarise the key issues in managing this patient.'*

Table 2.3 Post-clinic review.

Standard: 'Take me through each of your patients briefly. . . '
You may also want to summarise the patients you saw. You could offer trainees the opportunity to use one patient as a formal case-based discussion for their portfolio.
Mini-De-brief: 'How did the clinic go? Any concerns, difficulties? Which was the most interesting patient? Anything you need to follow up on before next time?'

- Give your own synopsis as a model.
- If the presentation seems unstructured, ask
  ○ *'What structure do you use for presenting patients?'*
- For more practice, ask students or junior trainees to go and write a summary, or a one-line synopsis, of patients they have seen and return later. You could give them a model to use.

To improve understanding and decision making
- Challenge learners to make sense of the information they have gathered,
  ○ *'How do you tie that all together physiologically?'*
  ○ *'What kind of processes do you think are going on?'*
- Clarify broad aims:
  ○ *'What are you trying to establish with your investigations?'*
  ○ *'What are your management aims?'*
- Ask for a rationale:
  ○ *'Explain why you would recommend not operating on this patient.'*
  ○ *'Why did you choose an ACE-inhibitor rather than a beta-blocker?'*
- Check clinical reasoning:
  ○ *'What other options did you consider and why did you rule them out?'*
  ○ *'What led you to conclude that this was a spurious result?'*
- Ask them to plan ahead:
  ○ *'How will you explain this to the patient?'*
  ○ *'What will you do if your plan does not work?'*

Other options
- Ask them to review the process they used in clerking:
  ○ *'What were the most useful questions you asked?'*
  ○ *'Was there anything else you should have considered?'*
- Ask them to consider the patient's perspective:
  ○ *'How do you think the patient felt at the end?'*
  ○ *'What are the implications for the patient's work?'*

Seeing the patient together
If, after the trainee has presented, you decide you need to see the patient for yourself, you may consider the following:
- Decide before going in who will lead the consultation. This may depend on a variety of factors, including whether the patient already knows you, whether you want to re-examine the patient yourself and how confident you feel in the trainee's ability to manage the consultation successfully.
- Think about where you sit as this will affect the dynamics of the consultation.

- Explain your role to the patient or ask the trainee to do so.
- If the trainee leads, you may still need to tell or ask the patient something, but try to avoid taking over.
- If you observe the trainee examining, you may also want to examine yourself, both to check their findings and to demonstrate your own examination technique.
- You can learn a lot about the trainee from observing him or her, and can review and give feedback afterwards.
- You could offer the trainee the opportunity to complete a Mini-CEx on the case.

Supervising students or trainees who are supernumerary:

Explain your practice
- Summarise the notes of the next patient to the learner as you are flicking through them and explain what you will be aiming to establish during the consultation.
- Explain why you do what you do (Box 2.10).
- Give practical hints from your experience:
  - *'Never help the patient undress because you can learn a lot from seeing how they do it.'*
  - *'I have a rule of thumb to spend twice as long with patients I find difficult.'*
- Explain what not to do as well as what to do.
  - *'Try to understand the whole history, not just treat the immediate problem.'*

Prompt observation
- After observing you during a consultation, ask what the learner noticed.
- Invite the learner to jot down any questions whilst you are seeing patients. Then, take a few minutes to discuss his or her notes.

Box 2.10 Making the invisible visible

A psychiatrist asked a patient with a history of drug use whether he was currently using. The patient said not and the psychiatrist turned to a different part of the history. Afterwards, he explained to the student that when he had asked the question he had also looked for signs that the patient was using drugs, such as dilated pupils and muscle twitching. His observations confirmed what the patient had said: hence, he had not questioned further.

- If you have two or more students in clinic, invite them to go for a coffee half way through, discuss what they have learnt and look up any information they need. Ask them to return with unanswered questions when they are ready. *This will allow them to talk through their impressions in a non-threatening way with someone at a similar level. By sharing and developing their knowledge in this way, there will probably be fewer, more focused questions for you.*
- Ask them to comment on the blood test/X-ray/ECG results. Include some that are normal as well as those that are not.
- Ask the learner to compare different presentations of the same diagnosis.
- Ask him or her to sketch out an algorithm for the investigation or management of patients with certain symptoms. You can check it later or ask them to compare it to the protocol.
- Look out for signs that the learner is flagging. To maintain motivation, change the activity, allow a break or release the student(s).

Set tasks
- Give observation/interpretation tasks to do whilst you are seeing patients:
  - *'Listen to the history and be ready to tell me the most important investigations you would request.'* This will encourage the trainee to listen more carefully and start to analyse the information.
  - *'Jot down your differential whilst I am taking the history and we will review it after the patient has left.'*

Box 2.11 A learning experience

A consultant explained and demonstrated some rehabilitation exercises to a patient, and got him to do them. During the next consultation, she asked the trainee to explain the exercises to the patient. The trainee showed the patient but did not ask him to demonstrate them. In the following consultation, the trainee's attention increased noticeably and later he had another opportunity to improve his explanation.

The consultant demonstrated good practice by getting the patient to demonstrate, not just watch the exercises. The trainee was not expecting to be asked to teach the patient and, although he had observed the previous consultation, had not fully appreciated the way in which the exercises had been taught. Advising learners that they will be applying something in the near future raises the level of attention and motivation.

- Encourage the learner(s) to summarise the notes for one or more subsequent patients. Depending on their level, you may give them time to
prepare this, whilst you see further patients:
  - *'Go outside and read the next patient's notes, and be ready to summarise
  them for me when I have seen this patient.'*
- Set an aim and give repeated practice (Box 2.11):
  - to examine the chest for each patient who requires it.
  - to interpret the ECG/X-ray or blood results for every patient.
- Allow time for learners to follow up issues (relevant to their level) whilst
you continue seeing patients:
  - *'Do you know what happens during a barium swallow?'* If the student says
  no, *'Go and look it up (or if possible, see it) and then you can explain it to
  the next patient who needs one.'*
- Set tasks for subsequent review:
  - *'Find out about the treatment of bowel cancer for Friday.'*
- If a separate room is available, ask the student(s) to clerk and present
patients – either individually, in pairs, or a mixture of both. *The advantage
of students working individually is that they get more skills practice, whereas
working in pairs allows them to share and compare ideas, articulate and
develop their thinking.*
- Ask the student(s) to write notes during the consultation as if for the patient record. At the end, they can compare their notes with yours. If good
enough, they could subsequently write the real notes for you to review.
- Ask the learner to draft the letter to the GP (taking time out from the
next patient). *This helps him or her to order information and consolidate
diagnostic reasoning and management planning.*
- Ask if the patient is able to stay an extra 15 minutes to tell the student/
trainee more about his or her daily life, impact of illness, community
care, etc.

General points
- You might aim for a mixed economy – the learner observing some consultations, taking part in others, doing some independently and undertaking
related tasks during others.
- At the end of the clinic, ask what gaps in the learners' knowledge have
been highlighted. Help them to specify what they need to learn, based on
what you would expect of someone at their stage. You may agree on some
'homework' to be reported back to you.
- Some departments have managed to negotiate 'teaching clinics' where
there are a reduced number of patients, allowing more time to discuss each
patient with their trainee/student.

Teaching in the Accident and Emergency department
This section highlights a few strategies that may be useful in the context of the Emergency department.

Individual review
Trainees: Depending on the stage of the trainee and how long he or she has been with you, you may wish to
• have every patient presented to you;
• see or discuss patients at the trainee's request;
• ask for random presentations;
• keep track of patient management online and check where plans are lacking or seem inappropriate.
Students: Ask students to clerk a patient, either individually or in pairs, and present to you or one of the team.

Students could keep a log of patients seen and management decisions made. They could follow up patient outcomes and present their findings back to the team.

Board rounds
At certain points, you may gather the junior doctors together around the board/screen containing the list of current patients and ask each to present. You can then draw out teaching points (see p. 26).

Options for board rounds
• Have set times when juniors know they will take place.
• Draw a proportion of the juniors together whilst others continue seeing patients. Then, swap. *This takes them out for less time, thus keeping patients moving through A&E better.*
• As above, but just take two of the team to see each other's presentations. *This increases their exposure to different cases whilst minimising service disruption.*
• Rather than asking everyone to present, ask only those who have an interesting case or questions to ask.
• Start with regular board rounds when trainees are new to the Department and gradually reduce the number as they become more competent.

A&E ward rounds
As for board rounds, but the trainees present in front of the patient.

Comments from Teachers *and Learners*

I find that what students always want is the hands-on practical.

I challenge students to be detectives, not reporters.

When I see follow-up patients that my trainees have operated on, I copy them into the letter, even if they have moved onto another placement: otherwise, they don't get the feedback they need.

I realised that I cannot teach the whole of the neurological examination in one session and that it is better to focus on one thing. That way, trainees come away feeling they have learnt something and can actually do something that is relevant and useful.

I tell students to assess every child's motor function and language – not just in clinic but at the bus stop or in the waiting room.

I like to give my juniors as much responsibility as they can manage and let them make as many clinical decisions as possible, so long as they know when to refer to me. I make sure that they know the criteria for discussing patients with me from the start of the placement, and understand that I want to see any patient they are unhappy with.

It would be fantastic to have a structure for how to report: to know what to leave in and what to take out.

I was very rarely asked after a clinic 'How did it go? Any questions?'

You feel silly if you are questioned in front of the patient and you don't know something because they know that you're a final year student, nearly ready to be a doctor and you feel embarrassed.

I think that the main thing I have learned from this consultant is how to manage the patients' expectations.

Teaching the interpretation of images/specimens

General principles

- People learn to interpret images by interpreting images! They need initial guidance, followed by lots of opportunities for practice and regular feedback.
- Encourage comparison between normal and abnormal images.
- Tailor the teaching and learning to the level of the student/trainee. For example, you might ask a student to identify a few common presentations, whilst an ST might be expected to describe the image according to a set structure and make a differential diagnosis.

Useful strategies

After taking a history and examining the clinical signs, you may then look at the patient's investigations such as the observation chart and imaging.

- Before looking at the image (or investigation/observation), ask:
  - ○ *'What are you looking for?'*
  - ○ *'What do you expect to see?'*

These questions help the student/trainee to think about the purpose of the imaging and combine observations with other clinical findings.

- Ask for comments on the image. Depending on the trainee's level, you might ask him or her to
  - ○ identify the type of image;
  - ○ name parts of the anatomy;
  - ○ describe the key features;
  - ○ identify whether normal or abnormal;
  - ○ point out any abnormalities;
  - ○ confirm/refute the provisional diagnosis;
  - ○ ask how the findings correlate with clinical signs and symptoms;
  - ○ evaluate the validity of the image.
- Ask what systematic approach he or she uses to interpret/report the image.
- Give a model answer to demonstrate what you expect.
- Ask the learner to describe the image in medical terminology to you and then in lay terminology to the patient.
- Ask for a justification of the interpretation.
- After hearing this, give your interpretation.
- After discussion, you could allow a second opportunity to present the findings. This gives the trainee/student an opportunity to consolidate learning and allows you to check his or her understanding.

Teaching in theatre

The operating theatre is a challenging environment for learning because aspiring surgeons and anaesthetists must develop their craft on real patients, observed by colleagues, often under pressure of time. Meanwhile, supervisors have to manage conflicting demands and interests, not purely practical but moral as well. As Atul Gawande says

> 'The moral burden of practicing on people is always with us but for the most part unspoken [. . .] In medicine, we have long faced a conflict between the imperative to give patients the best possible care and the need to provide novices with experience' [4].

Challenges identified by teachers in theatre include
- feeling under constant pressure from colleagues or managers to get through lists more quickly;
- finding it difficult to 'let go' of a patient, particularly with a new trainee;
- constantly wanting to take over when a trainee is working slowly or as soon as he or she runs into the slightest problem;
- worrying about being blamed, or even sued, for a mistake made by a trainee;
- feeling frustrated or bored when supervising rather than practically involved.

Thinking point

How many of the above apply to you?

Discussion

You may have felt most of them at some point. Some reflect the tensions inherent in a work environment where teaching is not the first priority. Others reflect the supervisor's responsibility for patient safety and it would be surprising (even dangerous) to be unconcerned about potential risks whilst watching a less experienced colleague operate/anaesthetise.

These difficulties have to be balanced against the responsibility to teach the next generation, and most people would agree that
- skills can only be learnt through repeated practice;
- trainees need to learn to find their own way out of mistakes (with or without guidance);

- safeguarding future patients means ensuring high standards of teaching now;
- theatre teams need to understand the importance of teaching and make reasonable allowances.

Ultimately, you have to make a judgement about when and how much to allow the trainee to do and when to take over.

Thinking point

What would make this judgement easier?

Discussion

Knowing what the trainee can do already is important, and this is much easier if you work together regularly. If not, it is worth discussing with trainees, colleagues and managers to see if there are creative ways to increase continuity. Alternatively, try some of the strategies listed on p. 51–52.

General principles

- Make expectations and rules clear. Do not assume that they are known.
- Experience is paramount, so give learners as much hands-on time as possible, relevant to their stage of training and within service constraints.
- Assess the trainee's existing skills and experience to help you judge how much he or she can do.
- Break skills into stages, and allow trainees to progress through them in a stepwise manner.
- Let them start slowly to stay safe and build confidence, and then gradually increase the level of demand and autonomy.
- Have trainees talk through the procedure with you before starting.
- Be aware of the stresses trainees face in learning under the constant surveillance of colleagues, and avoid making their mistakes more public than necessary.
- Take a few minutes to debrief after each patient and/or at the end of the list: this increases the value of learning.

Useful strategies

There are three stages to consider – before, during and after the trainee is in theatre. Sometimes, you may have more than one learner and have to consider how to involve them all (Box 2.12).

Box 2.12 Involving more than one trainee

Dr Jones, consultant anaesthetist, was in theatre with a registrar (ST5) and FY2 (Anne). She put the registrar in charge of the patient, and also asked him to explain various things to the FY2, such as how the oesophageal Doppler monitor is used. He checked if Anne had seen the machine before (she had not) and used a laminated diagram to describe how it works. Dr Jones then asked about factors affecting cardiac output and a discussion ensued in which Anne's knowledge was reviewed and important points elaborated. Later, Dr Jones discussed pulmonary artery catheters, getting the registrar to draw a graph and talk through it. She added further information and he brought up the text book graph on his mobile phone to check. She then gave Anne the patient's blood gases, asking what she would be looking for. Anne mentioned various factors and noted the patient's low sodium and high potassium. There was some discussion about how this should be managed. Dr Jones then gave the blood gases to the registrar, who discussed potential causes and management aims.

The following is a list of options from which to consider what might be appropriate in your situation:

Pre-operatively
Assess prior experience:
- Ask the trainee about similar procedures he or she has observed, assisted with or undertaken previously.
- Review his or her log book.
- Seek information from colleagues who have previously worked with the trainee (Box 2.13).

Encourage preparation:
- Check the trainee's knowledge of the patient. (Many surgeons and anaesthetists will not let anyone touch the patient who has not seen the patient before theatre).

Box 2.13 Monitoring progress

After a trainee successfully inserted an epidural into a patient, the Operating Department Practitioner (ODP) commented: 'That's 5/5 you have got in first time!' The anaesthetist realised that the ODP had had more continuity with the trainee than she had and thus a better knowledge of her progress.

- Ask the trainee to write out the steps of the procedure/operation before coming to theatre. This will help him or her to internalise it.
- Suggest trainees visualise the procedure in their mind before starting (some surgeons report doing this automatically).
- Refer the trainee to appropriate apps, for example, anatomy learning.
- Encourage trainees to make appropriate use of skills laboratories and simulation opportunities where available.
- If senior enough, allow the trainee time and space to prepare the list as he or she wishes.

Plan:
- Consider options for the practical involvement of the trainee(s):
  - Is it more useful to do one or more complete procedures or to practise the same part of the procedure on every patient?
  - Should a procedure be learnt in sequence from beginning to end? Alternatively, might trainees start with the simplest part and then proceed to more difficult parts?
  - Ask the trainee(s) how much/which part(s) of the operation they would like to do. They may know better than you what will help them – of course, you are not bound by this as you have other factors to consider.
- Discuss and agree who will do what before the list starts – whilst remaining flexible to respond to the situation as it unfolds. Where circumstances allow, this may be done a day or two in advance so trainees have time to prepare, and thus learning is enhanced.
- Ask the trainee when he or she would like you to scrub.
- Agree how you will indicate to the trainee that you want to take over, and vice versa, for example, 'I am ready now'. This is especially important if the patient is awake!
- Have the trainee talk you through the stages ahead and what he or she will do in the event of problems.
- Use diagrams or models as appropriate.
- Discuss whether the trainee wants to use the procedure for a PBA or DOPS.

Intra-operatively

Where learners are hands on:
- Ask them to talk you through what they are doing.
- Allow them silence in order to concentrate.
- Give practical guidance.
- Indicate alternative options.
- Clarify the overall aim as well as the immediate action required.

- Ask anaesthetic trainees to explain changes in readings on the monitors.
- Draw or have the learner draw relevant graphs or diagrams.
- Take photos or a video of the procedure for later review.
- Deal with extraneous issues to allow the trainee to concentrate.
- Have another trainee assist so that you can observe and take notes for later feedback.
- Stop and take over if necessary.

Non-verbal strategies:
These can be particularly helpful if a patient is conscious and can sometimes express things more easily than words. However, they may not always be appropriate, particularly if patient safety is at risk.

- Point to relevant equipment or anatomy.
- Use gestures to indicate how to do something or in which direction to go.
- Demonstrate without speaking.
- Indicate approval or disagreement non-verbally, for example, nod/shake of head, expression.
- Use gestures to indicate when to stop/start.

Where learners are observing in theatre:

- Check that they can see and invite them to move if not.
- Explain what you are doing and why.
- Ask them to identify anatomical features.
- Point out things to notice.
- Allow them to examine the patient.
- Ask if they can describe what you are doing.
- See if they can tell you the next stage in the process.
- Invite them to talk about previous similar procedures they have seen.
- Broaden the discussion (Box 2.14).
- Allow them to look up the procedure on the Internet whilst you are managing the patient, so that they can relate theory to practice.
- Ask other colleagues to explain their role.
- Involve them in small ways, for example, bringing the patient in, setting up equipment, checking medication, relaxing/distracting the patient, putting up drapes, recording observations, taking photographs and cutting sutures.

Post-operatively

Encourage patient follow-up:

- Allow the trainee to hand over the patient.

Box 2.14 Wider discussion

Whilst operating on a sebaceous cyst, the surgeon asked the trainee whether he thought it was related to the patient's hobby of horse riding. After discussing the cause, the surgeon described some technical aspects of the surgery. As the operation proceeded, the discussion moved onto veterinary practice (the nurse's dog had a sebaceous cyst), the ethics of cosmetic surgery, the psychology of patients seeking such surgery, post-operative complications (relating to a recent patient) and occupational diseases (the anaesthetist mentioned a recent text book).

- Involve the trainee in reviewing the patient before and potentially after discharge as well.
- Encourage him or her to follow up specimens in the laboratory.

Debriefing:
- Invite the trainee's thoughts through open questions such as '*How did it go today?*' or '*How did you find that?*' – then wait. Often trainees will start to evaluate their practice, ask questions or draw out learning points and future objectives.
- If appropriate, you could probe: '*What did you find most difficult? Anything you were unsure about? Anything you had approach differently next time?*
- Give direct feedback, including commenting on how they have progressed from previous cases and giving specific suggestions for development.

Further learning:
- If it was an interesting case, you might suggest that they use it for a reflective writing piece in their portfolio.
- To reinforce the procedure, get the trainee to write it out or draw a flowchart for you to check.
- Discuss the next stage of the trainee's development, identifying immediate and longer term aims.

'I am convinced that we must train not only the head, but the heart and hand as well.'

Madame Chiang Kai-shek, politician and first lady of China

Comments from Teachers *and Learners*

I try to absorb the stress of theatre so that the trainees can focus on what they're doing.

I find it useful to focus on one thing for the day. Sometimes, I get them to hold the mask so at the end of the day they know that they can now hold an airway.

I get my trainees to review the scans immediately after the operation, whilst the live view is fresh in their minds. This provides instant feedback and helps to develop their ability to interpret images.

We set up some scenarios, for example, putting faults into the anaesthetic machines and getting them to check it, or practicing the fire alarm with an anaesthetised patient.

Whilst I know that juniors are keen to perform as many operations as possible, I used to feel guilty if I left all the work to them – now, I have reconceptualised my role in theatre as 'educator' rather than 'clinician'.

In a procedure such as laparoscopy, I break down the steps into bite-size pieces and prompt the trainee to think about each one, such as what type of incision to make. It is important to slow down and analyse each step so that in time it becomes automatic.

They need practice but also feedback – without it, they can pick up bad habits.

It has taken me some time to accept that it is reasonable for trainees to learn during service provision and that, although they take longer than I would, they can still achieve a result that is acceptable to the patient.

I find it really difficult when I am trying to learn to intubate or put in an epidural and you've got the consultant behind you quizzing you on the physiology.

The learning curve tends to go up very sharply when you are allowed to make your own mistakes.

Good bosses will sit down at the end and tell you exactly what they thought you did well, what you need to do better and then follow that up with the next patient.

Some trainers do not bother to find out what you can do or are impatient and expect you to pick up skills instantly.

The most difficult thing is learning how to get yourself out of trouble because you don't have the experience. The bosses almost make it look easy because they are so practised, but it is a difficult skill to pass on.

Teaching practical skills

The main priority in teaching a practical skill is to ensure that it is learnt. This sounds obvious but is frequently ignored in practice. Have you ever been to a lecture on examining patients, breaking bad news or prescribing, where you are given lots of advice but no practice? Of course, it is possible to brief people on these areas but teachers are usually disappointed if they believe that telling someone how to do something equates to their being able to do it. The only way to ensure a skill has been learnt is to provide opportunities for practice and feedback.

A useful model for thinking about how skills are learnt is shown in Figure 2.2, which suggests four stages through which learners may progress.[2] To explore the stages in more detail, the example of learning to listen to heart sounds will be used.

Unconscious incompetence

At this stage, the learner is unable to perform the skill and is either unaware of it or does not understand its relevance or use. *So, imagine a student, 'Una'.*

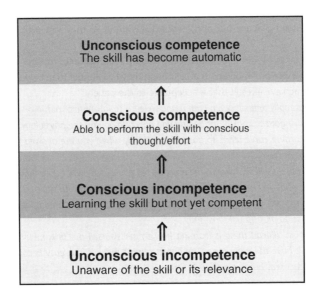

Figure 2.2 Conscious competence model.

---

[2] The origins of the model are unclear although Gordon Training International is widely recognised as influential in its development.

She is just starting medical school and whilst aware that doctors listen to the heart, she does not understand what they learn from it.

Conscious incompetence
The learner understands the need for the skill but is not yet able to perform it competently. *Following her physiology and pathology teaching, Una now understands why doctors listen for heart sounds. She is on her first medical firm, learning to use the stethoscope but having trouble discriminating sounds.*

Conscious competence
At this stage, the learner can perform the skill with conscious effort and thought. *Una is now in her final year and regularly listens to the heart. She makes a conscious effort to discriminate between sounds and can recognise some conditions.*

Unconscious competence
The skill has become automatic and the person no longer needs to think about what he or she is doing. *Una decided to become a cardiologist. Listening to heart sounds has become effortless and now she finds it difficult to understand why students struggle! She also finds it hard to explain what she is doing.*

Thinking point

Think of a skill that you teach and consider: What would help trainees to move from one stage to the next?

Discussion

To move from unconscious to conscious incompetence: you could describe and demonstrate the skill and explain how it benefits the patient. Alternatively, you could put learners in a position where they realise this for themselves. For example, if teaching about epidural injections, you could ask students to clerk a patient who needs an operation but cannot have a general anaesthetic because of a lung problem. Ask how they would resolve this problem, then let them watch the procedure and follow the patient into theatre and recovery.

Moving up the next two stages requires repeated practice and feedback. Sometimes, people may slip back a stage if they do not practise a skill for a while, or if a new technique or new equipment is introduced that requires further learning.

Skills are normally taught in a series of stages that help learners to progress, for example:

1. **Awareness**: ensuring that the learner understands the need for the skill and indications for its use.
2. **Observation**: demonstrating the skill (or ensuring that the learner has the opportunity to observe it).
3. **Supervised graduated practice**: (i) breaking the skill down into stages and deciding the order in which they should be taught (Table 2.4). Ideally this might be in a simulated environment initially, then on patients.
    (ii) Providing individual practice and giving detailed feedback on performance.
    (iii) Progressing to more difficult stages at the pace of the learner, and continuing to give feedback until the correct technique has been learnt.
4. **Remotely supervised practice**: facilitating further practice with guidance at hand. At this stage, the learner will continue to develop his or her competence, efficiency and ability to deal with problems.
5. **Independent practice**.

In many practical specialities, there are stipulated numbers of procedures that have to be undertaken and documented before trainees can progress from one stage to another. These provide a useful indication of the amount of experience a typical trainee may need to progress. Obviously, there will be individual variation, and the quality of supervision also makes a difference.

Table 2.4 Teaching a procedure in stages: an example.

Stages of tension-free mesh repair of an inguinal hernia:
1. Incision and initial dissection (incision placement and safe progression through layers of abdominal wall to reach inguinal canal and cord).
2. Dissection of cord and isolation of hernia sac (identification of direct or indirect defects, protection of cord structures, identification of ilioinguinal nerve and reduction/excision of hernia sac).
3. Placement of mesh (sizing of mesh, cutting to shape, inserting and suturing mesh and reformation of deep inguinal ring).
4. Haemostasis and closure (closing wound in anatomical layers).

Trainees might typically start on stage 4 which is the simplest, then progress to 1, then 3 or 2. Further subdivision can be made of each element. Each stage can be practised independently first (ideally several times within a day or week to cement learning) and then all in sequence.

Once able to perform all stages on easy cases, the trainee could progress to performing repairs under local anaesthetic, on larger inguinal-scrotal hernias and ultimately on emergency cases.

Table 2.5 Deliberative practice.[a]

It has traditionally been assumed that natural abilities account for the exceptional performance of individuals in a variety of fields such as sports, music and medicine. In fact, a plethora of studies have shown that sustained effort is necessary (but not sufficient) to reach expert performance and that the quantity and quality of practice is key.

A review of the acquisition and maintenance of skills found evidence for consistent gradual improvement when participants

1. were instructed to improve an aspect of performance of a well-defined task;
2. had ample opportunity to perform the same or similar tasks repeatedly.
3. received detailed, immediate feedback;

Performance increased as long as training sessions were limited to about an hour, as this allowed participants to maintain sufficient concentration to improve.

Many professionals reach stable levels of performance within a given time period, but those who become excellent, deliberately create or seek further opportunities for training at a higher level.

---

[a]Reference 5.

The development of practical skills can be accelerated by 'deliberative practice' (Table 2.5). Innovations such as simulation training or e-learning modules can clearly help to achieve the conditions for improvement, but how in theatre, clinic or on the ward could you help trainees to benefit from deliberative practice?

Thinking point

Look at the three conditions required for learning given in Table 2.5 and suggest ways of achieving them.

Discussion

You might consider the following:

1. Asking learners to identify a specific skill that they wish to improve or suggesting one that they need to improve, and clarifying what constitutes good practice. For example, when teaching trainees to use the ultrasound machine, you could ask them to locate the ovaries, demonstrating yourself on one side and then asking them to use the same technique on the other.
2. Focusing their practical experience on the specific goal and giving repeated practice, for example, asking them to locate the ovaries several more times on subsequent patients during the clinic.
3. Giving immediate feedback on what the student has done well, correcting errors and suggesting improvements. You might also prompt the student to evaluate his or her own performance.

Comments from Teachers *and Learners*

I let Harry do the radiotherapy planning first because he says he learns more from getting it wrong and being corrected than from watching me do it right.

Trainees may be nervous to do something in front of you in a way they have learned from another consultant because everyone has their own way of doing things. I try to re-assure them that that is ok so long as it is a safe technique and afterwards we can discuss the pros and cons of different methods.

It is repetition that is most important. Splitting tasks into smaller items can allow trainees to perform one thing multiple times but in perhaps slightly different operations – laparoscopic port placement in appendicectomy/cholecystectomy or bowel ops, for example, tends to be the same principles.

I think that simulations will become more important as our hours are reduced further, although it is difficult to get into laboratories that are good.

Detailed feedback whilst sitting with a drink afterwards is the best way to get learning points out whilst they are still fresh: this can then be practised in procedures later that day or week.

On-call/remote teaching

Doctors frequently give advice to junior colleagues over the telephone. So, how can you make this educational? A range of strategies are suggested from which you can choose those suitable for your situation.

Useful strategies

At the start

- Ring the trainee at the start of the shift, particularly if you have not met or worked together before. Let him or her know that you are available and how and when to call you.
- Ask about the trainee's speciality and level of training – this helps you to tailor your advice and gives you an idea of how much sleep you can expect!
- You could ask the trainee to specify at the start of each call whether he or she is seeking advice, asking you to come in or keeping you informed.
- Some supervisors like to give the trainee a structure for presenting the patient.

During the call

- Sometimes, giving straight advice is the best option, particularly if it is very busy or if you know that the trainee only seeks advice when he or she is really stuck.

- If you suspect that the trainee knows what to do but just wants reassurance, you could ask 'What are you thinking?' If you agree with the plan, he or she should gain in confidence.
- If the trainee presents information and then waits for you to take over, ask 'What do want from me?' This encourages him or her to formulate the problem, which is educational in itself.
- You could ask a question to prompt the trainee to think more broadly (Box 2.15).
- If the trainee asks a question, you could reflect it back:
  - *'What have you considered?'*
  - *'What are your options?'*
  Often, the trainee will come to a good decision by thinking it through with someone more senior. If not, you can say *'My approach would be . . .'*
- Give time limits and discuss contingency plans:
  - *'If he has not improved in the next hour, then . . .'*
- If you decide that you need to see the patient yourself, tell the trainee how long you will take to get there, whether you will be contactable en route and anything he or she needs to do in the interim.

Call me back instructions
- Clarify with the trainee when to call you back:
  - *'Call me again if the saturations go down/if you are worried.'*
- You could ask to be updated on the patient's progress within a particular timescale.

Box 2.15 A remote consultation

An ST2 working in critical care was called to see an 80-year-old lady with complications following a hip replacement. The patient had been given a prolonged course of penicillin following infection and now had a profound metabolic acidosis (base excess −15) and a rapid respiratory rate (40 per minute). Other signs were relatively normal and investigations unremarkable. The ST2 rang the on-call consultant, concerned about sepsis. The consultant thought this unlikely given the normal physiological and inflammatory parameters, and asked: *'What makes you think it is sepsis?'* The trainee paused and realised that the story did not completely fit. Thinking again, he said: *'She has been on paracetamol and fluclox for ages. . .'* The trainee realised that he had assumed sepsis because he was so used to seeing this in critical care, but the consultant's question had enabled him to stop, reconsider the wider picture and come to the right diagnosis of pyroglutamic acidosis.

Follow up
- Advise the trainee on any patients you think he or she needs to discuss in detail tomorrow/later, or with his or her clinical supervisor.
- Some teams have handover meetings where all the new patients are presented and discussed. Others have a nominated time in the week when queries from on-call shifts can be addressed.
- Find time to ask what the trainee learnt from the shift. He or she may like to use one or more cases, or the overall experience, for reflective writing.
- You might like to discuss and give feedback on the appropriateness trainees' calls. Avoid doing this when they first ring as it may deter them from making an important call, but you could discuss it when they report back, or the next time you see them.

The teacher who is indeed wise does not bid you to enter the house of his wisdom but rather leads you to the threshold of your mind.

Kahlil Gibran, author and poet

Teaching patients

Doctors have a central role in patient education and health promotion. The degree to which patients are informed and involved in decision making varies greatly, depending on the clinical context and on the views and preferences of individual doctors and patients. This may be a subject for discussion with learners who will also have their own views. This section contains ideas on how to educate patients from which you can select appropriately. There are many techniques which you can also use with learners.

Useful strategies
Check existing knowledge and concerns
- Check the record of what the patient has been told, but do not assume that he or she has necessarily understood or accepted the information.
- Find out what the patient already knows: *This will give you a starting point for your explanation and save unnecessary repetition.*
- Ask what the patient thinks is going on. *This may reveal misconceptions that you need to correct.*
- Ask about the patient's concerns. *This may save you having to give bad news if he or she already suspects it – you can confirm or refute the patient's suspicions and explain the next steps.*

• Ask if the patient would like someone else to be present during the consultation. *Another person may help the patient to remember information afterwards.*

Explain

• Remember that you talk about medical matters every day, whilst it may all be very new and unfamiliar to the patient.
• Explain what you know and what you do not know.
• Match your language to that of the patient: notice the vocabulary he or she uses and adjust your explanation accordingly.
• Show the patient his or her scans/results and explain what they mean.
• Try to pick up signals as to how much information the patient wants and can take. You might say:
  ○ '*I could go into more detail . . .* ' – and wait to see whether this is welcome.
  ○ '*Would you like me to explain the options or to make a plan for you?*'
• Explain what you intend to do next or offer choices.

Use props and aids

• Draw diagrams to aid your explanation.
• Use models, posters or computer images to illustrate what you say.
• Use everyday analogies to explain things in a way people can understand (Box 2.16).

Check understanding

• Pause after your explanation to allow time for information to sink in and questions to arise.
• Watch the patient carefully to gauge his or her understanding and emotional response to what you are saying.
• If the patient seems unsure about a decision, invite him or her to think about it and get back to you, or advise what to do if there is a change of mind.

Box 2.16 An unusual analogy

The heart is often described as a pump but Dr Said prefers a different analogy. She describes the heart as a house and explains how there may be problems with the doors (the valves), the electrics (the rhythm) or the plumbing – such as blockages in the pipes (the veins and arteries). She finds that this helps patients to understand that there may be more than one problem, with different treatments required for each.

Summarise
- Summarise what you have said and what has been agreed.
- Provide written information as backup (e.g., leaflets, copying the patient into your GP or referral letter). *Much of what was said will be quickly forgotten after you have left!*
- Give guidance on other sources of information, such as relevant websites and self-help groups, and, if possible, someone he or she can contact for further information.

Challenge

Think of any analogies you use or have heard others use. How effective are they? Think of concepts which patients find difficult to understand. Can you find any analogies that might help?

Discussion

Test your analogies on friends and colleagues and hone them to use with patients. Not all analogies work for everyone, so you may need more than one.

Teaching other disciplines

When teaching clinically, there may be other health care professionals present. Should you teach them, and if so, what and how?

Issues to consider
- Do they want or expect teaching from you? *Learning is more effective when it is sought and desired.*
- Are you working 1:1 or are there others with you? *Some non-medical colleagues may be reluctant to ask or be asked questions in front of other disciplines.*
- What should you teach? Consider the individual's interests, issues of immediate importance to a patient, areas where you notice or suspect a lack of understanding or topical issues relevant to his or her discipline.
- How much do they know? *As with all learners, this is a good starting point for teaching. You may want to find out more about their training and experience.*

Useful strategies
- Include relevant non-medical colleagues when gathering information about patients.
- Include them when you invite questions or leave space for questions to arise.

- Explain your actions or instructions where relevant to their role.
- Seek their views on issues relating to their areas of expertise – you may learn something and they will be more willing to ask you for information when the need occurs.
- When giving instructions, explain why they are important. If you fear that this may sound patronising, you could explain it to the patient in the colleague's presence.
- Encourage your trainees and students to exchange information with all members of the team.

Further reading on clinical teaching

McGee SR, Irby DM. Teaching in the outpatient clinic. Practical tips. *J Gen Intern Med* 1997; 12(S2):S34–S40. A summary of the evidence on learning in Outpatients, with detailed, practical guidance on specific strategies that can increase learning.

Ramani S, Leinster S. AMEE Guide no. 34: Teaching in the clinical environment. *Med Teach* 2008; 30:347–364. A summary of the major challenges facing clinical teachers in different environments, together with strategies and models that can be employed to enhance learning.

Lyon P. A model of teaching and learning in the operating theatre. *Med Educ* 2004; 38:1278–1287. A detailed study of the interpersonal dynamics in play in the operating theatre and how these influence opportunities for teaching and learning.

Bartleson JD. *How to be sure your patient education is educating patients.* http://beta.aan.com/globals/axon/assets/6106.pdf (accessed September 2013). A guide to the principles of and tactics for improving health education.

Dewhurst G. Time for change: teaching and learning on busy post-take ward rounds. *Clin Med* 2010; 10:231–234. Reporting trainees' perceptions of the learning opportunities on post-take ward rounds and how these can be integrated into practice.

Kennedy TJT, Lingard L, Ross Baker G, Kitchen L, Regehr G. Clinical oversight: conceptualizing the relationship between supervision and safety. *J Gen Intern Med* 2007; 22(8):1080–1084. A model of clinical supervision derived from an observational and interview study.

Royal College of Physicians, Royal College of Nursing. Ward rounds in medicine: principles for best practice. London: RCP, 2012. Guidance on restoring ward rounds to a place of central importance in caring for and communicating with patients.

References

[1] General Medical Council. *The Doctor as Teacher*. Manchester: General Medical Council; 1999.

[2] Agyris C and Schon D. *Organizational Learning: a theory of action perspective*. Reading, MA: Addison-Wesley Publishing Company; 1978.

[3] Bowen JL, Irby DM. Assessing Quality and Costs of Education in the Ambulatory Setting: A Review of the Literature. *Acad Med* 2002; 77(7):621–680.

[4] Gawande A. *Complications. A surgeon's notes on an imperfect science*. London: Profile Books; 2003, p. 23–24.

[5] Ericsson KA. Deliberate practice and the acquisition and maintenance of expert performance in medicine and related domains. *Acad Med* 2004; 79(10):S70–S81.

Chapter 3 **Workplace-based assessment and feedback**

The workplace-based assessments/supervised learning events

This section focuses on the tools currently used to assess and develop medical trainees' skills and knowledge. (For students, similar processes of observation and discussion of cases, followed by feedback, may be used.)

The majority of tools fall within three main categories which aim to explore different areas of practice (Table 3.1). The observation and discussion tools focus on single cases or occasions (and both can include assessment of the patient record), whilst the multi-source feedback (MSF) tools assess performance over time.

Several of the instruments were developed in North America and have been adapted for use in other countries. There is a growing evidence base for their validity, reliability and educational impact [1,2]. However, their value depends on the purpose for which they are employed and the manner and context in which they are applied.

They can be used in two main ways:

1. *formatively* (to provide feedback to learners about their performance and thus aid professional development);
2. *summatively* (to grade or rank individuals to inform decisions about their progression).

In the UK, the tools were initially introduced as 'workplace-based assessments' (WBAs). Trainees were required to complete a certain number and received grades and comments from supervisors, which were recorded in their portfolios. Whilst intended primarily to aid learning, they were often perceived by both trainees and supervisors as tick-box exercises [3].

How to Teach in Clinical Settings, First Edition. Mary Seabrook.
© 2014 John Wiley & Sons, Ltd. Published 2014 by John Wiley & Sons, Ltd.

Table 3.1 Categories of assessment/learning tools.

Method	Main areas assessed	Examples (see Appendix for glossary)	Description
Observational	Clinical skills	DOPS Mini-CEx ACE/Mini-ACE PBA OSAT	The trainee is observed interacting with a patient to assess clinical skills such as history taking, physical examination and practical procedures
Discussion-based	Clinical thinking and decision making	CbD ACAT	The trainee reviews a case or cases in which he or she has been involved so that the assessor can explore his or her clinical reasoning and decision making
Multi-source feedback	Professional behaviour	Mini-PAT MSF TO1/TO2 TAB SPRAT	Trainees rate themselves and ask a variety of colleagues or patients to rate them on set criteria relating to their professional behaviour. They review the results with a supervisor

In 2011, the General Medical Council proposed new terminology to clarify how the tools were being used, namely:

- supervised learning events (SLEs) when used to provide feedback (formatively);
- assessments of performance (AoPs) when used to determine progress (summatively) [4].

Since August 2012, the WBAs have been replaced by SLEs in the Foundation Programme. Gradings on the forms have been replaced with boxes to record qualitative feedback and trainees are advised that they are designed to help 'develop and improve their clinical and professional practice and to set targets for future achievements' [5]. The outcomes of SLEs will not be available at the Annual Review of Competence Progression, but the number undertaken is seen as a sign of engagement with the learning process. Similar developments in specialty training may follow, and evaluation will be required to see if the changes have the desired effect.

Using the tools effectively

The value of the tools for professional development is determined primarily by

- the nature of the discussion between trainee and supervisor;
- the quality of feedback provided (both verbal and written).

To be effective, both parties need to understand the purpose of the tools and commit the necessary time. If the process is perceived as form filling or a tick-box exercise, then almost certainly it will be so (Box 3.1). Time for clinical supervision and assessment should be built into job plans and agreed with clinical and management colleagues (see p. 92).

The following sections outline general principles and specific strategies relevant to some of the most commonly used tools, namely, the

- case-based discussion (CbD);
- directly observed procedural skills (DOPS);
- mini-clinical evaluation exercise (Mini-CEx) or mini-assessed clinical encounter (Mini-ACE) in psychiatry;
- multi-source feedback (MSF).

The teaching observation tool will also be considered because of its relevance to the content of this book.

General principles

- Your role is to help the trainees gain insight into their practice and set goals for development. This applies to all trainees, not just those who have underperformed in some way.

Box 3.1 Checking expectations

A consultant was conducting a case-based discussion with a fairly junior trainee. He sensed that the trainee was cynical about it and asked 'What has been your experience of CbDs in your previous rotations?' The trainee had not found them useful, feeling that they were just a formality to be got out of the way. The consultant said that he regularly had case-based discussions with colleagues and invariably found them informative. He put the form aside and asked the trainee to present the case, after which he led a discussion of the issues involved. He decided to leave completing the form until later as he did not want the trainee to be distracted from learning by his feelings over the marks he was given.

Table 3.2 Examples of agreed action.

To read Chapter 7 of Souhami and Moxham.
To research and produce a diagrammatic summary of the causes, presentation and treatment of renal failure.
To undertake two more supervised neurological examinations in the next week.
To sign and date every entry in the patients' notes (to be reviewed by random sample during ward rounds).
To observe the diabetic nurse's clinic to learn how to give advice on lifestyle and self-medication.
To undertake a specified e-learning module.
To present the patient at the next multi-disciplinary meeting.

- If you are an educational or named clinical supervisor, encourage trainees to link WBAs/SLEs to their learning objectives. For example, if they aim to improve their management of liver failure, suggest that they use a relevant case as a CbD.
- It is the trainee's responsibility to initiate the WBAs/SLEs. However, you can help by highlighting suitable opportunities and providing an environment in which the trainee feels able to ask.

Completing the forms
- Ask trainees to send you the form prospectively or, if not possible, immediately after the assessment: this facilitates timely feedback.
- Discuss your feedback with the trainee and then complete the form in his or her presence if possible.
- You do not need to grade or comment on every area on the form – just those you observe or discuss.
- Most of the forms contain an area for agreed action. It is usually best to invite the trainee to suggest learning goals first and then add your recommendations (see Table 3.2 for examples).
- There is sometimes confusion between 'areas requiring further work' (e.g. mental state examination or knowledge of diagnostic criteria) and 'action required' (e.g. supervised practice or specified reading).

Case-based discussion

Discussion of cases happens routinely in clinical work, and the CbD is just a way of recording these. The distinguishing feature is its focus on the clinical thinking employed by the trainee. It provides an opportunity to explore the decisions made appropriate to the trainee's level, for example, what was included in the initial assessment, the information given to the patient or the timing of the decision to call for senior advice. You may check whether the trainee has understood team decisions about the patient, but the main focus is on his or her contribution to care (Box 3.2).

Practicalities

- You can have some say over the case. You might negotiate which case the trainee will bring, or ask him or her to bring two or three cases, from which you choose one.
- Use a current or recent case so that it is relevant and memories are fresh: you could ask the trainee to bring a case at the end of clinic or after an on-call shift.
- Avoid making it a formal event. It is designed to be a discussion of work in progress, not a formal PowerPoint presentation.
- Trainees should bring the patient's notes, if possible, so that you can review their entries. This is particularly important if you do not know the patient so that you can check the accuracy of information given.
- Aim to elicit the trainee's thought processes and encourage his or her self-reflection. Table 3.3 gives generic questions suitable for most cases, from which you may select some to supplement more specific case-related questions.
- Sometimes 'why?' questions can promote a defensive response, so you may prefer to rephrase them, for example, '*What was in your mind when. . . ?*'
- The trainee should be doing most of the talking. Where this reveals gaps or misunderstandings, you can provide tailored teaching and advice.

Box 3.2 Differing perceptions

A consultant led a CbD in which she explored the trainee's management of a post-surgical case. She focused a lot of questions on the way in which the patient's fluid balance had been managed. At the end, the trainee commented that he had not really been involved in the patient's management. The consultant corrected him, reassuring him that his management had been what the patient needed.

Table 3.3 Generic questions for CbDs.

Why did you choose this case?
Give me a brief overview of the case.
What are the key issues in this case?
Explain your role in the case.
What are the key things to look for in a patient with . . . ?
What was the patient's main worry?
What did the patient think was going on?
How concerned were you about the patient?
What made you decide to . . . ?
What other options did you consider at that point?
What was your differential diagnosis?
How would you differentiate between x and y?
What did you expect (the investigation results) to show?
What did you surmise from the results?
What findings supported/refuted your provisional diagnosis?
What guidance/protocols/evidence did you use to guide you?
What contact did you have with relatives/other team members?
What ethical considerations were there in this case?
How well do you think you managed the case?
What did you learn from this case?
If you were to have a similar patient in future, what would you change?
What learning do you need to do as a result of this case? How will you do that?

Box 3.3 Use of CbD to review cases

Dr Aziz asks trainees who have made mistakes in a case but are unaware of it to use it as a formal CbD. He finds that during the discussion, they usually realise the errors they have made and he can then help them to develop an action plan to remedy shortcomings.

- Beware of spending too much time exploring the minutiae of a case: focus on exploring the trainee's understanding, drawing out learning points, correcting errors or misconceptions and planning future learning (Box 3.3).

This is general guidance, but expectations vary across specialties, so check your college website for specialty-specific information.

The mini-clinical evaluation exercise (Mini-ACE in psychiatry)

The *aim* of this tool is to evaluate how the trainee clerks a patient so that you can review and give feedback on history-taking, examination and communication skills. For this reason, you must *observe the trainee interacting with the patient*, not just listen to a case presentation. The insight that the observation provides will also help you to judge the level of supervision required by the trainee (Box 3.4).

Table 3.4 suggests areas you could focus on in your observations and Table 3.5 provides questions from which you can draw to prompt the trainee's self-review.

Practicalities

- Only fill in a Mini-CEx/Mini-ACE form if you have directly observed the trainee with the patient: if you are discussing a presented case, it is a CbD.
- These assessments may be best done during less busy on-calls, clinics or ward rounds, or on the A&E shop floor. You can take notes at the time and review them privately with the trainee afterwards.
- You do not need to observe a whole consultation. There will probably be plenty to comment on from just 5–6 minutes of observation.

Box 3.4 The danger of assumptions

Martin came into his ST4 placement with a reputation as a 'high flier' who had presented at national conferences and published research projects. Dr Weller was therefore surprised when, during a CbD, he had difficulty in identifying the key issues and got diverted down minor avenues. Subsequently, during a Mini-CEx, she observed that Martin did not give the patient enough time to speak and therefore missed important information. His record keeping also gave insufficient detail to allow for effective handover.

Dr Weller recalled that there had been previous occasions when supervising fairly senior trainees that she had noted concerns towards the end of a placement that would have been better dealt with earlier. She resolved to observe and assess new trainees early in the placement, explaining it to them as a matter of routine. This would allow any issues to be identified early and she could then step back for the latter part of their attachment.

Table 3.4 Suggested areas for observation and feedback.

The trainee's rapport with the patient.
Appropriateness of the questions asked.
Other questions you would have asked or other, more effective ways of phrasing them.
The sequence and technique of the examination.
Other things in the examination you would have included or done differently (you may want to demonstrate).
The clarity of his or her instructions and explanations to the patient.
The language used (whether appropriate to the patient).
Whether any cues were missed.
The appropriateness of the diagnosis and management plan.
The opportunity for the patient and relatives to ask questions.
How the consultation was brought to a close
The pace of the interaction and time taken.

Table 3.5 Sample questions to prompt trainees' self-review.

How do you feel your history taking/examination went?
Talk me through your thinking during the consultation. . .
What were you pleased with?
What was in your mind when you asked about . . . ?
Was there anything you were unhappy with or unsure about?
In retrospect, do you think that you could have phrased any of the questions better?
    (Give an example of a question that you think needed rewording.)
Was there anything else you should have included?
Did you have any problems eliciting signs?
What areas would you like to work on?
Alternatively, you could just ask one general open question such as 'How did that go?'

Directly observed procedural skills

Most supervisors find the DOPS one of the easiest tools to use because they are familiar and comfortable with supervising practical skills. However, there are a few issues that commonly arise, for example:

1. A trainee comes to you near the end of her placement saying that she still needs a DOPS to complete her portfolio. She reminds you that you saw her a couple of weeks ago cannulating a patient. Could you fill out a form for her?

2. You have seen your trainee catheterize a patient successfully and he now asks you to observe him again for a DOPS. This time he really struggles. At the end, he asks you not to submit the form (or he does not send it to you) as he was just unlucky this time – you know he can do it and he does not want a 'bad record'.

3. A trainee is known to be quite brusque with patients. You observe this during a DOPS and give him a borderline score. The trainee complains that he has always had good scores in previous DOPS.

Thinking point

Consider what you would do in each situation.

Discussion

1. The purpose of the DOPS (and all the tools) is to provide opportunities for reflection and feedback. It is unlikely that you can remember a case more than a couple of days ago in enough detail to give useful and accurate feedback. Do not feel obliged to fill in a form just because someone asks, but you may be able to offer another opportunity.

2. Trainees are often concerned about having anything even remotely critical recorded. Check your Royal College or Foundation School guidance for the latest policy on whether all assessments should be recorded. If do record it, you can advise the trainees that
   - you will give them an opportunity to repeat the DOPS before the end of the rotation: hopefully, this will show progression;
   - you will comment in the feedback that you have previously seen them perform the procedure successfully.

3. In the DOPS (and other observational tools), you assess the trainee on what you have seen. You cannot comment on other DOPS he has done but you can explain where he was below the standard required and what he needs to do in future to gain a satisfactory score.

In all of these situations, you have to make a judgement call. In wanting to maintain good relations with trainees, supervisors sometimes ignore or gloss over problems. Do not confuse the trainees' immediate concerns with their best interests. It is not your job always to be liked, and often the most respected supervisors are those who are able to address problems in an open and constructive manner. Be firm but fair. Judge trainees honestly and appropriately to their stage of training, give credit where it is due and help them plan how to address areas where improvements are needed.

Difficult situations can often be avoided if you advise the trainees early on in their placement about the purpose of and 'rules' for the WBAs/SLEs. These might include

- how and when they should negotiate with you to complete one of the tools;
- when they should send you the form to complete (normally prospectively);
- that it is their responsibility to complete the requisite number of tools in good time;
- that forms will not be completed retrospectively and that they should not request this;
- that they should ask a variety of colleagues to assess them;
- that the purpose of the tools is to aid their professional development;
- that they are only one part of the evidence used to recommend a trainee's progression, and are not used in selection to specialties.

It is helpful if teams can agree on ground rules so that everyone gives a consistent message.

Multi-source feedback (MSF)

The MSF is the only assessment in which you assess a trainee's performance as a whole, and anonymously. It requires trainees to seek feedback from a range of colleagues on their professional skills and attributes, such as teamwork and punctuality. If completed accurately and constructively, the MSF helps trainees understand how they are perceived by others, and compare that to their self-evaluation.

The educational supervisor would normally discuss the results of the MSF with trainees, acknowledging their strengths and helping them to formulate an action plan to address any areas highlighted as needing further development. If concerns have been raised, the supervisor may require trainees to repeat the MSF after a reasonable period and may select the assessors.

The following are examples of feedback given to trainees.

Good trainee – communicates well with patients.

Good team worker.

A few communication issues, but generally fine.

Needs to listen to colleagues more – does not always consider alternative views.

Enthusiastic about teaching.

Time management could be developed further.

Has had a few problems with patients. Too abrupt.

Needs to ensure explanation is understood by the patient.

Overall: approachable, professional. Works well with administrative staff and other health professionals.

Communication – sometimes perceived to be 'too upbeat' in certain situations.

Sometimes lacks confidence to take the lead.

Concerns re-time-keeping. Needs to improve reliability.

A safe doctor. Always punctual and works hard.

Challenge

Imagine that the above were written about you and consider which would be helpful (or not) and why. Then think of a colleague and write a few statements that would be honest and helpful in terms of motivating him or her to build on strengths and to address areas that need further development.

Discussion

Look at what you have written and notice how many are positive and how many are critical. Are they specific enough to be meaningful? If critical, are they framed as constructive suggestions for improvement? (See p. 81 for guidance on giving feedback.)

Comments from Teachers *and Learners*

When trainees ask me to do a Mini-CEx or DOPS, I ask them to make an appointment to discuss the feedback. Some of them just want to send the ticket, but I only fill it in if they come to see me because I am not interested in doing it just to get the box ticked.

I find CbDs more stimulating when you can go beyond the often routine choice of A over B and discuss wider issues such as decisions about when to stop treatment or how to tell patients when mistakes have been made, and how these make the trainee feel. These are areas that are not usually taught but must be developed before becoming a consultant.

I help the trainees to see the potential in any case. Some of them have gone on to do audits based on a CbD, or submit them as case reports to journals or as poster presentations at meetings.

We all have to accept that there are some rules and you just have to make time for the assessments.

I like to get the trainee to unpack a case and go back and review the decisions they made, considering what the alternatives were at each stage, and how the outcomes might have differed.

I am always interested in why the trainee has chosen a certain case – sometimes, it is because it challenged them clinically, or perhaps ethically and they are looking for reassurance. Sometimes, they just want to get good marks for their portfolio so they choose a case where they think they have excelled and then I might ask them to choose a different one.

The assessments are very useful because they force you to be formally observed and force the person observing to give formal feedback.

I found it more useful this year looking back at my assessment from the last Annual Review of Competence Progression and you can see where you have come from.

You have to meet the minimum requirements but the quality of learning depends on the trainee. You have to pin people down to help you – if you leave it late, it becomes tick-box exercise so the onus is on you.

Teaching observation tools

Tools are now available to assess teaching, and encouraging your trainees to use them demonstrates the importance you attach to their teaching. They tend to be used for formal presentations, but can also be used for clinical teaching – for many trainees, this is the only, or the most common, form of teaching they do. You do not necessarily need to see a whole session to comment.

The forms give you criteria on which to judge the teaching (see Table 3.6 for an example). Of course, these have to be interpreted, and the more knowledgeable you are about education, the better you can advise your trainees! You can also encourage them to gather feedback from learners (see Chapter 5).

Table 3.6 Descriptors of competencies demonstrated during teaching observation.

Introduction/gained group attention	• A formal or informal introduction as appropriate.
	• Ensures they have the full attention of the group before introducing the session.
Set out education objectives	• Objectives should be shared with the group and should be SMART based. They may be stated formally at the beginning of the session, or less formally as a general introduction. It is important that from the outset, the learners are clear about what is expected of them and what it is hoped they will achieve by the end.
Delivery	• Session has a clear beginning, middle and end. Topics and sub-topics are clearly linked together and placed into context. The session challenges but does not overwhelm the learners. There is clear development during the session moving from simpler material to more challenging concepts.
	• Key points are emphasised at various stages of the session, to assist learning and allow learners to prioritise the main messages.
	• Delivery is audible and learning points are understandable.
	• Learning environment managed effectively, ground rules are clear and seating arranged appropriately.

(continued overleaf)

Table 3.6 (continued)

Understanding of subject	• Facilitator displays knowledge appropriate to the subject matter and subject being taught.
Resources	• Teaching resources (slides/handouts, etc.) are used to support the teaching and are designed to meet the needs of the group being taught.
Effective group participation	• Appropriate interaction with the learners. Utilises different teaching strategies to maximise learning opportunities.
Teaching methods	• A range of teaching and learning strategies is utilised, such as small group teaching, role play and question and answer.
Feedback	• Assessment methods are clear from the outset. Feedback is given where appropriate.
Timing	• Session is delivered at an appropriate pace and facilitator's voice used to good effect.
Conclusion	• Clear summary of the main points of the session by facilitator or learners. Objectives revisited as appropriate.

Reproduced from www.jrcptb.org.uk with kind permission from the Joint Royal Colleges of Physicians Training Board [8].

Giving feedback

Tread softly because you tread on my dreams.

YB Yeats, poet
Quote suggested by a student recalling feedback received.

In this section, the focus is on giving feedback following WBAs/SLEs or during routine clinical supervision. There is further guidance on giving feedback during bedside teaching on p. 34.

Thinking point

Consider for a moment your own experience as a learner. Can you recall experiences of receiving helpful feedback? Think of specific examples and what made them helpful.

Discussion

Feedback is only effective when it is accepted and acted upon. It tends to be accepted when it is given by someone whom the learner respects, in an appropriate setting. It is effective when learners gain insight into specific aspects of their practice and use this to improve.

Giving negative feedback

This is one of the most commonly requested areas for advice. Some people object to the term *negative feedback*, and indeed, it has negative connotations because many people are reluctant to give such feedback. On the other hand, the terms *areas for improvement* or *development* can be seen as politically correct. What is less contentious is that learners want (and need) honest feedback that helps them to improve their practice: yet in student surveys, the provision of feedback is frequently one of the lowest-rated criteria.

So what deters people from giving negative feedback? Reasons include
- not knowing how to give it in a way that it will be accepted and valued;
- concerns about being accused of bullying;
- worries that learners will get upset.

The good news is that you can learn to give feedback – of all shades – effectively and to feel comfortable, even enjoy the process!

Thinking point

Before moving on to consider principles and models of feedback, take a moment to reflect on any transferable skills you may have. Think of situations inside and outside medicine in which you have given difficult information or corrected others in a way that proved effective.

Discussion

Most doctors have broken bad news to a patient at some point. How did you learn to do that? Can you use similar techniques with learners? Or have you been involved in sports coaching, music tuition or bringing up children? If so, what approaches to feedback have been effective?

The following sections suggest some general principles and structures to help you become more effective at giving feedback.

General principles of feedback
- Your intention counts: a genuine desire to help transmits itself.
- Reframe *negative* feedback to *developmental* feedback (feedback to aid the learner's development) in your mind: then you will find it easier to give.
- Think of feedback as a dialogue: you are providing information with the hope that learners will act on it, so you need to keep them with you.
- Provide balance: reinforce what was done well alongside discussing goals for development.
- Prioritise key points – or just one key point. Give the amount of feedback the learner can use, rather than that which you are capable of giving.
- Notice how individuals respond and adapt your feedback style accordingly: some people are motivated by reassurance, others like to be corrected.
- Try to get agreement on the issues quickly so that you can focus on solutions.
- Treat feedback as a normal part of work.

Useful strategies for giving feedback

Before you start
- Try to gauge if your feedback is welcome: if not (for whatever reason), then it is less likely that your suggestions will be acted upon.
- Build rapport: aim to establish a good relationship with the learner before giving feedback.

Prompt self-evaluation
- It is usually helpful to elicit learners' self-evaluation first: this helps you to tailor your feedback appropriately.
- If an error has been made, try to help learners to realise it themselves: this is usually more powerful than telling them. Ask questions that help them to recognize what they have missed and understand the implications:
  - ○ 'What happened to the patient's blood pressure at the moment of knife on skin?' [Asked where a trainee had not observed this.]
  - ○ 'How much did the patient know about the diagnosis already? How would it have helped you to know that?'
- Another option is to make a factual observation and invite the trainee's response (Box 3.5).
- Or give your opinion or impression, and wait for the trainee's comment:
  - ○ 'I have noticed that you are more slick with your examination now. . . '
  - ○ 'I sensed that you were struggling a bit with the differential diagnosis. . . '
- Sometimes, it helps to prompt the learner to see things from someone else's point of view:
  - ○ 'Why do you think that the radiologist did not accept your referral?'
  - ○ 'Put yourself in the patient's position. How do you think that she would have described you?'

Explain or demonstrate
- Often it is best to start with positive feedback but there may be times, for example, when there has been an obvious problem, that you might deal with that first, and then return to more positive aspects.

Box 3.5 Feedback on professional behaviour

A trainee was due to see a patient in the community clinic. She did not arrive on time and the consultant asked the receptionist to ring and check where she was. She was en route and arrived 10 minutes later. After the clinic, the consultant invited questions on anything from the clinic, and then commented 'You were not here at the start of the clinic and you did not let us know . . . .?' The trainee apologized and explained how she had finished the morning clinic late because she found it hard to bring consultations to an end and get the notes written up in the allotted time. They discussed different ways of concluding consultations, and the consultant emphasized the importance of making contact if delay was unavoidable so that the receptionist could inform the patient and colleagues.

Box 3.6 Examination skills feedback

An FY2 asked a student to examine the patient's abdomen and present his findings. She observed, and then said 'This is how I do it.' She demonstrated her own examination technique and presented her findings, which were slightly different to those of the trainee.

Comment: When observing the trainee, the FY2 noticed some errors but did not correct them in front of the patient. Rather she allowed the trainee to observe and work them out for himself.

- You could show, rather than tell the learner, what should have been done (Box 3.6).
- Sometimes, it may be better to give small bites of feedback as the learner is examining/performing a procedure, rather than all at the end.
- Be specific in your comments so that learners understand the criteria against which you are assessing their performance:
  - ○ 'Your explanation was thorough and you used simple, non-medical language which the patient seemed to understand. You also recorded the consultation in an appropriate level of detail.'
- If there is an issue which the learner seems unable to recognize, then you need to explain. Describe the unwanted behaviour in a neutral way, giving examples or evidence. Then explain the behaviour the learner needs to demonstrate and why it is important.
  - ○ 'I have had feedback that you are not making yourself available to juniors for advice. This is important because it is part of your role to support them in the same way that I am available for you. If you cannot respond immediately, then explain why and give them a timescale in which you will get back to them.'

Plan action points
- Prompt the learners to suggest their own ways to improve:
  - ○ 'How could you improve your ECG interpretation?'
  - ○ 'What do you think could help you to run the clinic more efficiently?'
- Encourage them to commit to goals and changes in practice, for example,
  - ○ to go through the e-learning module on ECG interpretation by the end of the month;
  - ○ to dictate letters after each patient rather than at the end of the clinic next week.

- If the learner does not accept the feedback, it may be a good idea to give some thinking time – for both of you! You could arrange to meet again in a few days (probably not more than a week), by which time, the learner may have had time to reflect and accept the feedback. In the mean time, you could discuss with your colleagues how to approach the situation.

Feedback models and structures

Contrary to popular opinion, there is more than one effective way to give feedback! Often people are taught either the 'Pendelton's Rules' or the 'Sandwich Model' as gospel. Each of them has strengths and weaknesses and there are other options too. An evidence-based model of how to structure the feedback conversation is given in Figure 3.1.

Pendleton's rules

These were proposed as rules for giving feedback about consultations and have been widely adopted for feedback in general. A four part structure was suggested, namely,

1. clarifying matters of fact;
2. encouraging the learner to go first;
3. considering what has been done well first;
4. making recommendations for improvement, rather than stating weaknesses [6].

Sandwich model

This is the positive/negative/positive structure. You comment first on the positives, both to acknowledge and reinforce good practice and to avoid the defensiveness that might arise if you went straight to the negative aspects. You then comment on what did not work so well and end on a positive.

These two models can be effective in certain situations. Both identify positive aspects, which can easily be forgotten in the rush to correct! Pendleton's asks for the trainee's view first, encouraging reflection against specific criteria and allowing the supervisor to judge the trainee's insight. Positive aspects are then reviewed. Finally, improvements are recommended: the wording is positive, unlike in the Sandwich model, and avoids the implication that such areas are inherent weaknesses. This is a safe model, which can be useful if giving feedback to someone you do not know well.

If used too often or too rigidly, both models can become formulaic and irritate trainees. If using them frequently, try to vary the wording, so for example, when discussing potential improvements you could ask 'What would you do differently?' 'What would you change another time?' or

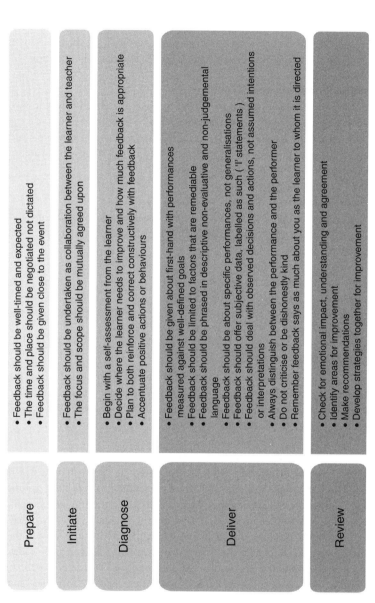

Prepare
- Feedback should be well-timed and expected
- The time and place should be negotiated not dictated
- Feedback should be given close to the event

Initiate
- Feedback should be undertaken as collaboration between the learner and teacher
- The focus and scope should be mutually agreed upon

Diagnose
- Begin with a self-assessment from the learner
- Decide where the learner needs to improve and how much feedback is appropriate
- Plan to both reinforce and correct constructively with feedback
- Accentuate positive actions or behaviours

Deliver
- Feedback should be given about first-hand with performances measured against well-defined goals
- Feedback should be limited to factors that are remediable
- Feedback should be phrased in descriptive non-evaluative and non-judgemental language
- Feedback should be about specific performances, not generalisations
- Feedback should offer subjective data, labelled as such ('I' statements)
- Feedback should deal with observed decisions and actions, not assumed intentions or interpretations
- Always distinguish between the performance and the performer
- Do not criticise or be dishonestly kind
- Remember feedback says as much about you as the learner to whom it is directed

Review
- Check for emotional impact, understanding and agreement
- Identify areas for improvement
- Make recommendations
- Develop strategies together for improvement

Figure 3.1 Structuring the feedback conversation [7]. Reproduced with permission from Strachan SR (2013).

'Imagine that you see a similar patient tomorrow: how would you manage her?'

Both models polarize thought into what has or has not gone well, rather than, for example, exploring what happened and why. Other options include:

Chronological approach

Ask the trainee to talk you through the event in the order in which it occurred: *'So how did you plan the anaesthetic? How did the induction go? What happened next?...'*

Usually, this will encourage the trainee to reflect on his or her rationale and comment on concerns or issues which arose. You can then discuss the issues raised, adding your own feedback as appropriate.

This method can promote a thorough evaluation of the trainee's work. It may take longer than other methods and therefore be difficult to achieve if time is limited.

Criteria-based approach

In this method, both you and the trainees are aware of the criteria that will be used to judge their work. These may be pre-set (as on the CbD/Mini-CEx forms) or agreed before the evaluation. You then go through each of the criteria, with you or the trainees commenting as appropriate. The WBAs/SLEs lend themselves to this kind of approach as the criteria are explicit, and trainees are expecting feedback.

This provides a clear structure, known by both parties before the observation. It can be useful for examination practice where the assessment criteria are available or where you have been asked to check specific things that the learner finds challenging.

One minute feedback

You tell the learner: 'One thing I liked was . . . , one thing to work on is . . . '
It is important to be specific, for example,

'One thing I liked was the structure of your history: you elicited the information in a logical way and covered all the main areas. One thing to work on is developing your formulation: practice summarizing each case in a few sentences giving your overall impression and differential diagnosis.'

This is quick, so may be suitable for bedside teaching, and can work well in a group setting as everyone is treated in the same way.

Open or trainee-centred model
You encourage the trainee to comment by asking a neutral, open question, such as '*So . . . ?*' or '*What do you think?*' and then wait. Alternatively, you could ask '*What would you like to gain from our discussion?*' You then respond to the issues he or she raises, for example, by asking further questions, explaining or giving information, recommending resources or discussing action points.

This is less judgemental, allowing trainees to set the agenda to a greater degree and raise issues that are important to them. However, issues that you think are important could be missed if the trainees do not recognize them.

In reality, you can mix and match aspects of different models according to what you think will be most effective in any given situation.

Example of feedback options

> A patient develops an infection following a procedure conducted by your registrar. Colleagues report that the registrar was not thorough enough in her preparation and there were deficiencies in her aseptic technique.

Depending on the registrar's attitude and insight when you ask her to review the case, you could take one of following approaches (which start gently and become more assertive):

- Turn the criticism into a constructive suggestion: 'Always remember to think through potential complications before you start and be scrupulous about asepsis.'
- Or, more strongly: 'Next time, think through potential complications in detail and document the steps you are taking to prevent them.'
- Alternatively, you could ask a series of questions to help the learner to reflect on his or her practice:
  'What potential complications did you consider before starting?
  Were there others you might have considered? (Explain if necessary.)
  How well do you think you prepared for these? How did you prepare?
  Describe the principles of asepsis.
  What steps will you take with a similar patient next time?
  What is the evidence for your approach?'

This approach can be effective with unreflective trainees as it makes them come up with the answers for themselves.

- If you feel that you need to make it stronger still, you could tell the trainee: 'I will supervise you next time you do this procedure and check your technique.'
  'This is what you need to do in future if I am going to sign you off: . . . '
  'I will be checking over the next few weeks to make sure that you do x, y and z. . . '

Final thought

Awareness of a range of strategies and models can be helpful, but at the end of the day, feedback is just another interaction between two human beings. Sometimes, listening carefully to the trainee and following your instinct about what and how much to say is the best policy. Seeing someone improve as the result of your feedback can be one of the most rewarding aspects of teaching.

Comments from Teachers *and Learners*

Do not give feedback when you are in a bad mood. Have a cold beer first!

Most people know their deficiencies and are relieved when someone actually flags it up.

Sometimes, it is quite awkward if consultants ask you to highlight your strengths and weaknesses. My concern is that I will have no insight and look even worse!

Further reading on assessment and feedback

Academy of Royal Medical Colleges. *Improving assessment*. London: AMRC. 2009. An informative report reviewing the introduction of workplace assessments across medical colleges. It includes appendices summarising the evidence for effectiveness of the most commonly used tools.

Chowdhury RR, Kalu G. Learning to give feedback in medical education. *Obstetrician & Gynaecologist* 2004; 6 (4):243–237.

Norcini JJ. *Workplace-based assessment in clinical training*. Edinburgh: ASME. 2007.

Nicol DJ, Macfarlane-Dick D. Formative assessment and self-regulated learning: A model and seven principles of good feedback. *Stud High Educ* 2006; 31:199–218. A useful, evidence-based model.

See individual Royal College and Foundation School websites for up-to-date information on requirements and current tools.

References

[1] Norcini JJ. *Workplace-based assessment in clinical training*. Edinburgh: ASME; 2007.

[2] Academy of Royal Medical Colleges (AMRC). *Improving assessment*. London: Academy of Royal Medical Colleges; 2009.

[3] Academy of Royal Medical Colleges (AMRC). *Improving assessment*. London: Academy of Royal Medical Colleges; 2009. p 8.

[4] General Medical Council. Learning and assessment in the clinical environment: the way forward. 2001. Discussion document downloaded from www.gmc-uk.org [accessed on 21 July 2013].

[5] AMRC, The UK Foundation Programme Office. Supervised learning events (SLEs). Frequently asked questions (FAQs). Downloaded from www.foundation programme.nhs.uk [accessed on 21 July 2013].

[6] Pendleton D, Schofield T, Tate P, Havelock P. *The new consultation. Developing doctor-patient communication.* Oxford: Oxford University Press; 2003. p 77. (This reviews the original recommendations and comments on their use and misuse.)

[7] Strachan SR. Unpublished MA thesis. University of Dundee; 2013.

[8] Joint Royal Colleges of Physicians Training Board. www.jrcptb.org.uk [accessed on 21 July 2013].

Chapter 4 **Common problems in clinical teaching**

This chapter is devoted to issues and concerns that commonly arise during courses on teaching.

Balancing teaching and service demands

Time is usually the biggest constraint on teaching whilst providing a service to patients. When working in a busy clinical area, it can be easy to prioritise service provision and miss teaching opportunities. However, health care providers receive substantial recompense for teaching and therefore doctors should not feel guilty about taking time to teach: in fact, it is a core responsibility [1].

Thinking point

1. Do you know how much your trust/practice receives for teaching?
2. Do you know how much students pay for their medical training?

Discussion

Funding for medical education is too complex to be described fully here (and is constantly evolving). However, a few components are worth noting because substantial sums are involved, yet teachers are often unaware of them.

1. **The Service Increment for Teaching (SIFT)**: Trusts and general practices receive this payment, which is designed to compensate them for the excess service costs incurred because of teaching undergraduates – for example, the fact that clinics and theatre lists will take longer when students are involved.

How to Teach in Clinical Settings, First Edition. Mary Seabrook.
© 2014 John Wiley & Sons, Ltd. Published 2014 by John Wiley & Sons, Ltd.

Trainees' salary costs: Secondary care providers receive payment to deliver postgraduate medical training programmes.
Table 4.1 gives further details.

2. **Tuition fees**: In the UK, students pay annual tuition fees, except for Scottish/EU students studying in Scotland. In 2012–2013, fees for clinically based programmes for home/EU students were mostly £9,000 per annum. Overseas students pay about three times as much: for example, in 2012–2013, Imperial College London charged £39,100, Cardiff £26,500 and Edinburgh £34,850.

Table 4.1 Financial support for training placements.

Service Increment for Teaching (SIFT) funding
The following examples gives an indication of the figures involved:
- SIFT payments for NHS trusts in London amounted to £320 million according to the London Deanery in 2013 [2].
- The Warrington & Halton hospitals NHS trust received £593,000 in 2009–2010 for their contribution to teaching medical students from the University of Liverpool [3].
- The East of England 'Stage 1' placement fee for four students spending eight days in general practice from 2010 to 2015 is £6,640 [4].

Trainees' salary payments [5]
Historically, funding was calculated to reflect the proportion of time which it was assumed that trainees contributed to service. For Foundation Year 1: 100% of basic salary was paid (i.e. assuming no contribution to service) + £2,000 non-pay costs. For Foundation Year 2 and Speciality Training Years 1 and 2: 50% of basic salary and for Speciality Training Year 3 and above: 100% of basic salary was paid, plus £2,800 non-pay costs.

New arrangements [6,7]
The previous arrangements are being replaced by a tariff system in which medical placements in secondary care are funded as follows:
Undergraduate: £34,623 (from April 2013).
Postgraduate: 50% of trainees' basic salary plus a placement fee of £12,400 (from April 2014).
Both tariffs will be adjusted by the 'market forces factor' and there are arrangements to ease the transition from the previous system.

Useful strategies
- Try to ensure that your teaching responsibilities are fully recognised in your job plan: there may be local guidelines specifying how much time should be allocated for different educational roles [8].

- If you have a wider remit (Head of Department, College Tutor, Training Programme Director), you could raise teaching issues at a higher level and champion, for example, dedicated training lists or clinics with time for teaching built in. It may be worth finding out what colleagues in other specialities have achieved: there is often considerable variation.

That said, there will always be time pressures, so the following strategies may help to maximise learning with time limits:

- Focus your teaching on certain patients: consider which will provide the best learning opportunities. Tell the learners that you will teach on this/these patient(s), and they can observe you manage the others, asking questions if they wish.
- Be opportunistic: sometimes there are fewer patients on the ward, or patients who do not attend clinic. Use these times for teaching, and learners will be more understanding when things are busy.
- Remind learners at the start of a clinic, list or ward round that this is a learning opportunity! In practice, teaching and learning is happening all the time during routine work, but is not always recognised as such. It is surprising how differently the occasion can be viewed by learners if this is made explicit.
- Focus on what cannot be learnt from books. Help learners work through a clinical case rather than quizzing them on factual information. *Clinical reasoning is best learnt from an experienced clinician, whereas facts are relatively easy to find independently.*
- Prioritise: Assess your learners' weaker areas and focus on them.
- Work as a teaching team. Think who is best equipped to teach, and delegate. Often learners find that the person one stage up the ladder from them is most attuned to what they need.
- Give small bites/chunks of information.
- Give yourself a target time to devote to teaching and divide it appropriately.
- Aim to convey one learning point for each patient.

Also remember that you may not be teaching, but students can still be learning, so think about creating an environment in which learning can take place (Chapter 1). Earlier sections of the book contain many strategies which involve students and trainees working independently and then reviewing their work with you: this increases the value of the time they spend with you.

Good teachers are costly, but bad teachers cost more.

Bob Talbert, journalist

Pitching teaching at the right level

One of the most frequently asked questions on teaching courses is how to determine the level at which to teach.

Thinking point

1. Three students arrive, saying that they have been timetabled to join your ward round. How can you assess their level in the couple of minutes before the ward round starts?
2. You have a new registrar due to run a parallel clinic with you next week. How do you know how closely to supervise her?

Discussion

The above decisions depend on knowing the current level of the individual or group. So, before you start, find out about the learners' relevant experience and knowledge. This is known as undertaking a 'learning needs assessment' or you could think about it as taking an educational history.

Many years ago, Ausubel stated

> The most important single factor influencing learning is what the learner already knows. Ascertain this and teach him accordingly [9].

If you are an educational or named clinical supervisor, much of your initial meeting with the trainee may be taken up with exploring his or her prior knowledge and experience. In a clinical setting, it can be done very quickly (2–3 min). Just a few questions can give you the information you need to start to make an educational diagnosis and plan (Tables 4.2 and 4.3).

Useful strategies

Depending on the time available, you might choose from the following:
- If you know that the learner(s) are coming beforehand, then find out about their stage of training and level of experience.
- Ask colleagues who have previously worked with the learner(s) for their opinion.
- Ask the learner(s) about areas such as
  ○ previous experience of the context in which you are teaching;
  ○ previous teaching/supervision they have received;
  ○ their concerns and expectations;
  ○ their aims for the session.

Table 4.2 Sample assessment of student before first clinic.

What kind of clinics have you attended previously?
What involvement did you have?
What do you hope to learn here?
Which conditions are you expecting to see?
How would you like to be involved in the clinic?

Table 4.3 Sample assessment of ST4 before first clinic.

- Tell me about your previous experience of clinics.
- What level of supervision did you have?
- How confident do you feel about this clinic?
- Are there any areas you are concerned about?
- What kind of supervision would you prefer? [Note: you are responsible for determining the level of supervision but it may be helpful to get the trainee's view first.]

- You might also want to ask some factual or procedural questions to establish their level of knowledge more precisely:
  - *'What do you know about cancer staging?'*
  - *'Talk me through the main stages of the mini-mental state examination.'*
- Watch them examine a patient or carry out a practical procedure – there are few better ways to get a feel for an individual's ability than to see what they do in practice – however, be aware that they may be nervous and therefore not perform at their best.

Teacher's comment

I always ask people where they went to school because then I know whether they understand how services are organised in the UK.

Dealing with complaints and clinical incidents

Imagine that you have a trainee who has recently started with you. He has been on nights for the first week and today you have received a complaint from a nurse about his handling of a case. You are told that he ignored nurses' suggestions and waited too long before calling for senior advice.

General principles
- Be straightforward about the fact that there has been a complaint/clinical incident and that you need to review it with him in order to learn from it.
- Consider the timing – is it better to deal with the incident straight away or to wait? If the trainee is exhausted or upset, he may need time to absorb what has happened and come to terms with it. However, if you wait too long, memories will fade and important lessons may be lost. If you decide not to debrief straight away, then arrange a time very shortly afterwards.
- Acknowledge the trainee's feelings. If you have had a similar experience, it can help to mention this, without getting side tracked into a detailed discussion of your experience.
- If the incident is one of a series of concerns about the trainee, it may be helpful to ask a colleague who was not involved in the case to sit in on the discussion (perhaps the Training Programme Director).

Approaches to the review
In reviewing the case, there are two broad approaches:
1. **Encourage self-reflection**: Help the trainee to analyse his or her practice in order to learn what went wrong and how to act in future (see next section). Helping trainees to work this out for themselves is often more effective than telling them because they develop insight.
2. **Give feedback**: This is useful if time is short or if the trainee does not recognise his or her errors or misconceptions. For effective ways of giving feedback, see Chapter 3.
Often the two approaches are combined – you can encourage trainees to review their own practice and then give feedback on any areas that they have not addressed, have misunderstood or of which they are unaware.

Encouraging reflection

Kolb's model of experiential learning (learning from experience) can be applied to facilitate trainees' self-review (Figure 4.1) [10]. In this model, you act as a facilitator rather than a teacher, asking questions to help the trainee reflect on the case, rather than giving advice or a lecture. The model has four stages, each of which will be described, referring to the above case to illustrate how it could be applied.

1. **Concrete experience**: the experience on which the person will reflect. *You could ask the trainee to describe what happened on the night in question.*
2. **Critical reflection**: the process of reflecting on the case and its impact. *You could ask how the trainee was feeling at the time and how he or she now views the events.*
3. **Abstract conceptualisation**: identifying relevant principles, theories or evidence. *You could prompt the trainee to review the decisions he or she made, analyzing the consequences and considering other options that were available at the time. If a lack of knowledge is identified, that could lead to generating some learning objectives. You might also prompt the trainee to consider wider factors contributing to the situation, for example, having been on nights during the first week in a new placement. There may be things that you or senior colleagues also need to address.*
4. **Active experimentation**: planning future approaches. *You could ask how the trainee would deal with the same situation if it happened again. This would help him or her to rehearse a more effective strategy. (This may take place at a later stage after information has been researched following stage 3).*

Supervisors who have tried this method are often surprised by how well trainees can work out their own solutions. In the short term, it may take time; however, in the long term, it can save time by preventing future errors. You can direct the trainee's thinking by the questions you ask, and if necessary give advice at the end.

Other options and strategies are as follows:
- Ask the trainee to write a reflection on the case and review with you.
- Prepare him or her for any necessary paperwork or meetings regarding the incident.

Having heard the trainees' account, you need to consider the seriousness of the case:
- Is this a one-off or part of a pattern? (You may want to seek others' views.)
- Were they just unlucky? – It could be, but beware of jumping to this conclusion too quickly just because it makes life easier for you!

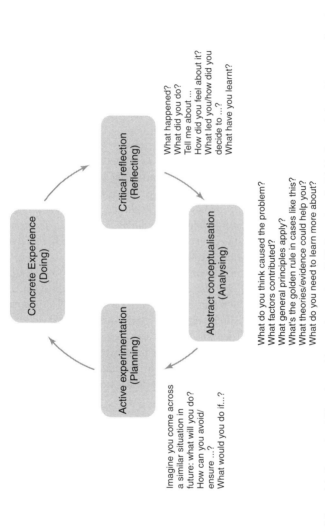

Figure 4.1 Kolb's model of experiential learning, with sample questions [10]. Reproduced with kind permission of Pearson Education, Inc., Upper Saddle River, NJ.

Table 4.4 Sample letter following review of a communication problem.

Dear xx

Thanks for coming to discuss the recent case with me. I appreciate that it is difficult to receive a complaint, but it was helpful to identify the reasons for it, which should help you to avoid such situations in the future.

We discussed how you felt that the patient had misinterpreted your comments, how you might pick up on this in future and the need to check back with patients about what they have understood.

We agreed that you will do two Mini-CExs with consultants within the next month and also observe the nurse practitioner with a patient who has received bad news. We will review these when you come for your mid-placement review meeting.

- Does it have implications for their training? For example, do they need further training in certain areas? If they are on a recognised training programme, are there implications for their progression? – If so, with whom do you need to discuss this?
- Are there implications for their current role? Do they need to be removed from certain duties or given greater supervision? Who else needs to be informed?
- How is your discussion to be recorded? (e.g. e-mail, letter or minutes of meeting). This is particularly important if you feel that there are wider issues – either because the trust/practice may view it as a serious incident or if it is someone who has already been identified as a 'trainee in difficulty'. You should record the nature of your discussion and any agreed action points (Table 4.4).

Teacher's comment

At HEMS [Helicopter Emergency Medical Service], we debrief after every single incident and it is all written down. Colleagues also shadow each other and give feedback.

It is important to involve other colleagues at an early stage so it does not become 'personal' and perceived as bullying – this often happens in my experience – so asking others to 'assess' the trainee early on can help avoid that.

Ad hoc teaching

Two students approach you asking for teaching whilst you are busy on the ward. What do you do? Options include the following:

- Invite them to shadow you and ask questions as you go along.
- Engage them in helping you with your jobs in return for some discussion about the patients (take blood pressure/temperature, check observation chart, look up something in the BNF [British National Formulary], dipstick urine, take blood/blood gases, help with line/tube/drain insertion).
- Explain that you are busy now and suggest another time when you would be willing to teach.
- Ask what they are looking for (their learning objectives) and then decide whether you can provide that now or later.
- Suggest a task that they can do now (e.g. clerk a patient or review some X-rays) and arrange a time they can return to present their findings.
- Ask them to go on a 'patient journey' (accompany the patient to radiology/ physiotherapy/occupational health/swallow assessment/cardiac investigation etc.), then report back on what they observed/learnt.
- If on the Intensive Treatment Unit/High Dependency Unit, ask the student to make observations from the end of the bed about the support patients are receiving (intravenous lines/infusions/monitoring/ventilation/protection of pressure sites etc.). They can report these to you on the spot, or on your return 5–10 min later.
- Ask them to check a patient's drug chart and let you know what medication is prescribed regularly/occasionally/one-off/route of administration, any drug allergies, etc. – then discuss with them the clinical indications for the medications given.
- Ask them to look at patients' observation charts and surmise whether the patient is improving or deteriorating.

What you choose may depend on the time and patients available, or you could offer a choice. In an ideal situation, the students would come with something specific they want to learn/practise and you could accommodate it. In real life, they may not have thought about what they want and will need to fit around what is feasible for you. Aim to engage them actively, either in practical ways or in interpreting/thinking/planning/observing/researching and reporting back to you.

Teaching people at different levels together

During ward rounds and sometimes in clinics or theatre, you may have several learners at different levels within the same group.

Some general principles are as follows:
- Aim to establish an environment where everyone feels able to contribute or ask questions without feeling foolish.
- Try to include everyone in one way or another.
- Maintain the credibility of senior members of the team in front of more junior trainees and students.
- Foster a teaching ethos by encouraging the team to ask and answer each others' questions and work together for the good of the patient.

Useful strategies include the following:
- Vary who presents cases or interprets investigations, allowing each person to have a turn (Box 4.1).
- Ask questions which are not reliant on knowledge where everyone can have an opinion, for example, about an ethical issue.
- Engage the whole group in joint problem solving, allowing everyone to find their own way to contribute.
- Ask open questions to the whole group and let whoever wishes answer.
- Graduate your questions so that more senior trainees answer more demanding questions.
- Invite more senior trainees/students to teach more junior ones.
- Allow several people to answer the same question at different levels.
- Direct certain explanations/information to specific team members relevant to their role.

Box 4.1 Involving the team

A consultant led a ward round with three male and one female trainee who was pregnant at the time. As he discussed the patients, he asked questions of the male trainees but not the female. When asked about this afterwards, he said that pregnancy was tiring and he did not want to stress the trainee any further.

Whilst the consultant's intention was positive, it was open to misinterpretation by the trainee. She felt that since becoming pregnant, she was often discounted by colleagues and worried that her career would be adversely affected.

- Aim to discover and draw on individuals' specialised knowledge, for example, students who have done a BSc or individuals who have worked in another country or specialised unit.
- If someone answers incorrectly, seek other views.
- Ask occasional questions to which you do not know the answer to demonstrate that you do not 'know it all' – encourage discussion of possible answers and perhaps a strategy for investigation.

The true aim of every one who aspires to be a teacher should be, not to impart his own opinions, but to kindle minds.

FW Robertson, preacher

Teaching older or more experienced colleagues

There may be situations in which you feel unqualified to teach or feel you lack the authority to do so, for example, some new consultants find themselves teaching former peers who have not progressed as quickly. You may also have staff grades and trust doctors reporting to you who have a wealth of experience. The following approaches could be considered:

- Value your colleagues' experience whilst recognising that you are in your position for a reason.
- Stick to your areas of expertise.
- Offer a professional discussion.
  - ○ *'If you want another opinion on any of the patients, just ask.'*
- Be open to learning yourself and confident enough to acknowledge that you can learn from junior colleagues.
- Ask for others' opinions: this demonstrates respect for their views. Then, you can either agree or give your own opinion and explain why it differs.
- Be clear about which decisions are yours, and if you are ultimately responsible for patient care, you need to take the final decision, even if it means agreeing to disagree.
  - ○ *'I appreciate that there are different views about how to manage this kind of patient, but for patients under my care, I always/I prefer to . . . '*
- Explain your decisions without being defensive.
  - ○ *'The way I approach this is . . . '*
- It may be best to avoid pushing yourself as a teacher. Aim to earn your colleagues' trust and confidence (e.g. through maintaining high standards in your own practice) and they will come to you.

Teacher's comment

Some of the registrars can be slightly overconfident and I have to make a conscious effort not to be press-ganged into doing things their way. At the same time, I don't want to curb their enthusiasm so I try to listen to them and discuss their ideas.

Engaging the quiet or reluctant learner

Doctors often express difficulties in teaching 'quiet' students or trainees – wondering whether to involve them, and if so, how. Some, afraid of provoking upset, pass over the quiet students and focus their attention on those eager to contribute. Others take a sink or swim attitude, forcing reluctant students to contribute despite their obvious embarrassment. It is probably best to aim for a middle way!

General principles
Include all students in discussions and practical activities: *all need to learn (Box 4.2)*.
Give equal eye contact to all.
Encourage rather than force: *this will build rather than destroy confidence.*
Be aware of cultural factors. *Some learners brought up in other cultures may be used to a more didactic style of teaching and take time to adapt.*

Useful strategies

During discussions/questioning
- Vary your tone: ask the question in a more gentle way.
- Allow prior preparation:
  - *'Tonight I want you to look up the causes of hypercalcaemia and I will ask you tomorrow.'*
  - *'Once I have assessed the patient, I am going to ask you to tell me what you have observed about her.'*
- Alternatively, give more time to answer, for example, if they do not answer quickly, say *'I will come back to you in a minute.'*
- Ask an open question *(where there is less likelihood of the student getting a wrong answer)*:
  - *'What do you observe about the MRI (magnetic resonance imaging) scan?'*
  - *'Tell me any investigations you might consider.'*

Box 4.2 Learning through teaching

A registrar was teaching some fifth year students about the examination of the acute abdomen. Shortly afterwards, a group of third year students arrived and she asked the fifth year students to teach them the same skill. She felt that this consolidated their knowledge, whilst allowing her to check their learning.

- Ask about experience or opinion rather than knowledge, for example,
  - *'What would be your preferred antibiotic?'*
  - *'How have they approached this in other places you have worked?'*
- Ask them to look up something, for example, a drug dose or something in the patient's notes.
- Allow them to discuss with a colleague first, for example, ask students to compare there differential diagnoses and then present to you. *This reduces anxiety as it allows them to check ideas before making them public.*
- Ask if they agree/disagree or would like to add anything to what has been said.
- Invite them to ask you a question: *'Is there anything you would like to ask or clarify?'*
- Tell them *'I do not expect you to know this, but . . . ?'*

If after trying some of the above strategies, you still feel uncomfortable, ask the quiet person privately outside the group whether he or she is happy to be included in your questioning.

Practical involvement (e.g. examining patients)
- Divide tasks into small stages.
- Give reluctant students shorter or easier tasks at first if you think that they lack confidence.
- Explain that everyone will have a turn and ask who would like to go next.
- Ask students to decide themselves the order in which people contribute. They may know each other better than you do and will be sensitive to their peers.
- Keep the tone positive and encouraging.

The difficult consultation

Paula had been suffering from severe back pain for some time that was inhibiting her life and work. She was referred to a surgeon but was very anxious about having surgery. At outpatients, the surgeon (observed by two students) assessed her and immediately told her that she needed surgery. Paula was upset by the prospect and felt that he had not listened to her concerns. She told him 'You don't listen to me', and started crying.

You will sometimes encounter difficult situations with a patient or relative whilst accompanied by trainees or students – and they can learn a lot from seeing how you handle such situations. However, if things do not go well, you and the learners may feel embarrassed. So, how can you turn such an event into a learning opportunity?

- Ask for the learners' ideas:
  - *'How would you have handled that situation?'*
  (*Not*, 'How do you think I did?') *It is rarely helpful to ask learners to critique your performance because, as a teacher, you are in a position of power. It puts them in a difficult position and is unlikely to elicit honest feedback. If you want genuine feedback, it is better to ask the patient or a colleague of similar or greater seniority.*
- Draw on the learners' experience:
  - *'How have you seen other people deal with similar situations?'*
- Be honest about your feelings:
  - *'I did not handle that very well.'*
  - *'I found myself feeling quite angry with the patient.'*
  Acknowledging your failings can help trainees feel able to admit theirs too. However, beware of becoming confessional and looking to the learners to make you feel better. Establish the issues you need to work on and move on.
- Give your own evaluation and lessons learnt:
  - *'I think that I jumped in too soon. Another time I would try to introduce the idea more slowly, maybe ask if the GP has told them about possible surgical options.'*
- Lighten the mood: *'Right – I've shown you how not to do it!'*
- Draw out general principles:
  - *'So, what principles apply when dealing with patients who are upset?'*

Teaching multiple students

What can you do if the group of students is too big to take on a ward round or into clinic?

Useful strategies include the following:

- Stagger them: divide into smaller groups and timetable them on different days. Or, preferably, get them to organise the timetable themselves, giving them details of the learning opportunities and maximum numbers for each.

- Rotate them: have a variety of activities around which the students work in groups of two or three. For example, with a group of eight, two might be in outpatients, two in endoscopy and four in pairs, clerking patients for presentation at the weekly teaching meeting. In subsequent weeks, they swap roles.

- Share them amongst your team. Students could be divided into pairs and allocated to different colleagues, each asked to address a topic from the students' curriculum. On subsequent days, the pairs rotate around.

- Allocate students to willing patients, and have them take detailed notes of the patient's medical history and treatment. The students could then research the relevant medical condition(s), meet up to share their learning and experience or write them up as case studies.

- On a ward round, the group might divide into two, each half accompanying the team for half the round. Subsequently, they could read around issues identified during teaching and then follow up the patients over the next few days.

- In clinics, pairs of students could work in turn to clerk and present a patient to you and then go and write a summary or draft letter to the GP.

- Rather than going into theatre, students could watch operations via a live link to a teaching room.

Teaching trainees with no interest in your speciality

Perhaps the trainee is not interested in your speciality *yet*. He or she may never be – but many trainees have been attracted to a speciality by an enthusiastic teacher, and even those who think that they know their destination early on can change their minds.

Whatever their career intentions, every speciality has something to offer to every trainee.

Useful strategies
- Show interest in the trainee's preferred speciality and what attracts him or her to it.
- Draw links between your speciality and his or her preferred choice.
- Encourage the trainee to identify ways in which knowledge gained in your placement could be useful in his or her intended speciality (Box 4.3).
- Identify and prioritise skills that could be useful in either speciality.
- Ask what the trainee thinks he or she can contribute to your patients.
- Explain that he or she will learn the referral criteria for your speciality.
- Focus on the patients' needs and their right to good care from everyone involved.
- Inspire by your own enthusiasm and example.
- Suggest additional opportunities for learning that relate directly to the trainee's interests.
- Give examples of things you learnt in other specialities that you did not realise until later would be relevant to your own.
- Take a problem-based approach – most trainees are motivated by having problems to solve.

Box 4.3 Making the links

Salim, a GP trainee on a hospital rotation, presented a patient with Crohn's disease to his consultant physician. The consultant asked: 'What would you do if this patient had presented in general practice?' Later, he suggested that Salim made a point of thinking about how a GP would follow up such cases. He recommended some reading and explained why it was relevant to general practice. He also suggested that Salim asked about similar patients next time he was at the practice.

Teacher's comments

Because most medical students do not become psychiatrists, I am very aware of what psychiatry they need to be FY1s. So, they have a log book in which they summarise, say their schizophrenia patient's history, and then a section where they consider what the issues would be if that person was in a medical or surgical ward under their care. So, get them to extrapolate to different settings relevant to their learning needs.

Luke's motivation increased sharply when I asked him to chair the multi-disciplinary meeting and he has since taken a lot more responsibility for discharge planning.

References

[1] General Medical Council. *Good medical practice*. England and Wales, Scotland: GMC; 2006.

[2] www.londondeanery.ac.uk/undergraduate [accessed on 19 July 2013].

[3] http://www.whatdotheyknow.com/request/medical_students_sift_payments [accessed on 19 July 2013].

[4] www.medschl.cam.ac.uk/Intranet2/students/az/documents/GP-Pro-rata _Agreement_10-15_RD.pdf [accessed on 19 July 2013].

[5] Department of Health. Introduction of tariffs for education and training. Impact Assessment No. 8050 MEF. 2013.

[6] Ibid.

[7] www.dh.gov.uk/health/2013/02/implementation-tariffs/ [accessed on 19 July 2013].

[8] Some deaneries had their own guidelines, for example, www.nwpgmd.nhs.uk /educator-development/standards-guidance/job-planning [accessed on 19 July 2013].

[9] Ausubel, DP *Educational psychology: a cognitive view*. New York: Holt, Rinehart and Winston Inc.; 1968.

[10] Kolb, DA. *Experiential learning: experience as the source of learning and development*. Englewood Cliffs, NJ: Prentice-Hall, Inc.; 1984.

Chapter 5 **Next steps**

> I long to accomplish a great and noble task, but it is my chief duty to accomplish small tasks as if they were great and noble.
>
> *Helen Keller, deafblind author*

Developing as a teacher

As with most skills, the more proficient you become, the more you will tend to enjoy teaching. Teaching skills are also in demand – frequently asked about at interviews for speciality selection and consultant posts. Sometimes candidates are even asked to undertake a short teaching session as part of the selection process. There are also opportunities to develop teaching as a career interest, with a range of educational roles and positions available.

This chapter provides ideas as to how you can further develop your teaching, including sections on self-evaluation, gathering feedback from learners and useful resources.

Ways to develop your teaching

- Be creative: try new ideas and approaches to teaching and see how they work.
- Increase your knowledge of educational theory by reading or undertaking relevant e-learning (see resources section).
- Talk about teaching with your peers. Tell them about your experiences and seek their ideas on areas you find difficult.
- Learn more about your students' and trainees' programmes. Get to know your local undergraduate and postgraduate leads and ask them about new

How to Teach in Clinical Settings, First Edition. Mary Seabrook.
© 2014 John Wiley & Sons, Ltd. Published 2014 by John Wiley & Sons, Ltd.

developments. Access medical school and Royal College websites to find their curricula containing course objectives and assessments.

- Experiment with technology to aid your teaching – learn to use the interactive whiteboard (smart board) or computerised voting systems (if available locally), or design an on-line learning aid. Also remember traditional but still useful teaching aids such as flipcharts and whiteboards.
- Keep a log of your teaching. Have a dedicated document or journal in which to note down things that worked, ideas of how you might address problems or new things to try. It can be interesting to look back on these ideas as you develop your teaching.
- Notice what other teachers (medical or non-medical) are doing around you in the clinical environment. Can you apply any of their successful techniques?
- Join a teaching group (either local or national) and attend relevant conferences.
- Become an examiner. It is a good way to get feedback on training and to identify areas which students/trainees need to develop.
- Volunteer for an extra role within the medical school or postgraduate centre. Usually, you will be made very welcome – particularly in dedicated teaching environments such as the clinical skills centre or simulation suite.
- Apply for a formal teaching position. Depending on your level of experience, you could take responsibility for co-ordinating an area of teaching within your unit or medical school.
- Find a colleague (or learner) who is also interested in teaching and develop a project together – a new course, a new assessment method or perhaps undertake a small research project.

Evaluating your teaching

How do you know if you are teaching well? There are a few ways to find it out:

Self-evaluation

Notice what does and does not work. You may find a certain diagram that is effective in explaining a difficult concept, or a particular question that prompts trainees to apply theoretical knowledge to practice. Pay attention to verbal and non-verbal cues – when do learners seem most/least interested and engaged? If you have a really successful session, take a few minutes to jot down what worked and consider how you can use these methods in future.

Consider the balance of your interaction with learners. If you are talking for 80–90% of the time, then you are probably also doing most of the thinking. Try to redress the balance and elicit learners' views and plans: this allows them to practise weighing up information and making decisions under your supervision.

Thinking point

Look at the statements in Table 5.1 – which apply to you? If there are any that do not, consider what you could do to encourage them.

Table 5.1 Signs that your teaching is effective.

Learners ask questions without needing to be invited – *this shows that they are thinking and that you are approachable*
They tell you about their previous experiences, what they have read and what they think
They admit to weaknesses or mistakes
They improve their knowledge and skills – you notice progression in their clinical work
They show enthusiasm for and commitment to their work, for example, attending regularly and maybe staying longer than expected
They engage in teaching others
They ask you for more teaching!

Discussion

You could try the direct approach and ask for these things to happen, but a more effective way would be to create an environment in which they happen naturally (see Chapter 1).

Peer evaluation

Ask a colleague to attend your teaching and give you feedback. The choice of colleague is important here – you need someone you respect, who is a good teacher and who you trust to provide a constructive critique. You may like to get more than one opinion and you might consider including non-medical colleagues who will focus on the teaching methods rather than content. Some medical schools and colleges have education advisors who offer teaching observations.

Video/audio recording

In some situations, with permission from those involved, it may be valuable to record teaching for your own review. If you do this, it can be useful to review the recordings with someone else. Most people are not used to seeing/hearing themselves, and it is easy to focus on things which do not matter much to others, such as small mannerisms which do not inhibit learning.

Feedback from learners

Asking learners for feedback can be helpful in order to give you qualitative information about the effectiveness of your approach. You could use a form or seek verbal feedback.

How not to do it: Do not ask '*Was that alright?*' It is a leading question, and most learners will be far too polite to disagree, especially if you are more senior than them or likely to assess them.

Similarly, do not ask '*What did not you like?*' – again, it can put learners in a difficult position and may also be quite negative for you. You could ask specific questions such as '*What was most/least helpful?*', '*Is there anything I should leave out/add in?*' or '*What do you think would be the best way to teach this subject?*' These all encourage comments which will help you to improve your teaching.

How to collect feedback

Plan

- Consider what you hope to learn from the feedback. Do you want to know whether the learners enjoyed it? What they learnt? How you could improve it? How your teaching compares to others'? Whether it was the right topic?
- Then, plan how you can obtain this information. If using feedback forms, consider whether ratings or comments will be most helpful. Ratings can give you a general impression of how much the students liked your teaching, which aspects of teaching they found more or less helpful or how your session rated compared to others (if you all use the same form). Comments can give you information about what students learnt, what specifically they found helpful and why, and how you can improve.
- Sometimes you might prefer to give trainees an open forum or blank sheet to comment on anything they want to, rather than pre-determining the questions. This may give you different information.
- Decide whether you want feedback on a specific teaching event, on your teaching in general or both.
- Decide if you will offer the opportunity for anonymous feedback or whether you prefer learners to own their feedback.
- Plan who will collect and collate the feedback (you, the students or a secretary), or if verbal feedback, how it will be recorded.
- Plan when will you ask for feedback – during a placement (when learners may benefit from actions taken as a result) or afterwards (when they may be more frank) or ideally, both.

Collect the data

- Have an open discussion with learners about what they have learnt so far, what they find difficult and how you could adapt your teaching to help them.
- Ask a colleague to have a discussion with learners about their experiences and report back to you.
- If you have a group, you could nominate one person to collect feedback from his or her peers and present to you
- Give out individual feedback forms for either single sessions or a group of sessions - e.g. all teaching in outpatients (see sample questions to draw from in Table 5.2).
- Post an on-line feedback form.

Collate, interpret and act

- The interpretation of evaluation data is down to you. Avoid giving too much weight to individual comments, although sometimes these can be very informative.
- Consider making changes suggested by students, or other ways in which you can address any concerns.
- Evolve your teaching by experimenting with new ideas and re-evaluating.

Programme or placement evaluation

If you are responsible for a programme or placement, you may wish to collect feedback on the trainees' overall experience. Some commonly used formats with sample questions are given in Table 5.3, or you could hold a meeting to discuss learners' experiences.

You could organise joint meetings of teachers and learners in order to discuss issues from either side. Alternatively, you can disseminate the feedback you have gathered to teaching colleagues and discuss the results at a meeting.

And finally, remember to keep examples of evaluations as evidence of the steps you have taken to develop your teaching. These may be needed for re-accreditation but can also be interesting as a record of your own evolution as a teacher.

Table 5.2 Sample questions for feedback forms.

What has helped you to learn in clinic/ward round/theatre?
What was most helpful and why?
What would increase your learning?
What would you like to do more of, less of?
What learning will you take away?
How could the supervision/teaching be improved?

Table 5.3 Options and sample questions for collecting feedback on clinical placements.

Rating Scales

How would you rate the following (on a scale from very good – very poor):
* the quality of supervision?
* availability of staff to supervise?
* the induction programme?
* the formal teaching programme?
* the placement overall?

Opinion statements (on a scale from strongly disagree to strongly agree)
I was given constructive feedback on my work.
The aims and objectives of the placement were clear.
I felt supported by the clinical team.
I was clear about how I would be assessed.

Qualitative Feedback

Please comment on the following areas:
* the timetable (e.g. workload, variety of experience and learning opportunities)
* the induction (quality of information and integration into team)
* supervision arrangements (e.g. availability of supervisors, opportunity to present cases)
* teaching (e.g. quality of teaching, provision of feedback)

What did you value most about this placement?
What would improve the placement?

If you do things well, do them better. Be daring, be first, be different, be just.

Anita Roddick, businesswoman and campaigner

Useful resources

Courses

Junior doctors are increasingly expected to attend short teaching courses and, as they advance, training in assessment and supervision. Clinical and educational supervisors are required to be appropriately trained and to undertake continuing professional development for these roles. Doctors applying for educational posts within medicine increasingly have a formal educational qualification.

There are many courses available, varying from short half- or one-day courses to accredited Masters programmes taking several years. Courses may be run by Royal Colleges, deaneries (or their successors), health care trusts, postgraduate centres of teaching hospitals, universities, further education colleges or medical education organisations. Look at the relevant websites to find out more.

Masters programmes are offered usually in three stages – the certificate and diploma, typically taking a year each, followed by a research project in the final year. Some programmes are specifically for doctors, others for health professionals and some are multi-faculty. The format also varies: some are available as distance learning packages (which may be helpful for trainees moving around placements or unsure where they will be working in future) and others require regular attendance or a residential component. If you are interested in developing the teaching side of your career, consider your preferences and ideally speak to others who have completed such courses. Your local postgraduate centre should be a good place for initial enquiries. Bursaries are sometimes available.

Recommended books

Newble D, Cannon R. *A handbook for medical teachers*. Dordrecht: Kluwer Academic Publishers; 2001. *A very readable dip into type book with lots of suggestions geared to medical teaching and assessment.*

Ramsden P. *Learning to teach in higher education*. Oxon: Routledge Falmer; 2003. *An excellent review and discussion of educational research findings with practical examples – a book that may change the way you think about teaching and learning.*

Dobson S, Bromley L, Dobson M. *How to teach: a handbook for clinicians*. Oxford: OUP; 2011. *Useful advice on planning teaching, including simulation, and an interesting appendix on language issues in teaching. Also contains resources for those wishing to run workshops on teaching including sample course programmes and handouts.*

Gibbs G, Habershaw. *Preparing to teach: an introduction to effective teaching in higher education*. Bristol: Technical & Educational Services Ltd.; 1992. *An accessible introduction to teaching, giving practical advice on areas such as lecturing, teaching small groups, labs and practicals and supervising projects.*

Cantillon P, Hutchinson L, Wood D (eds). *ABC of learning and teaching in medicine*. London: BMJ Publishing Groups; 2003. *A series of articles on teaching and assessment in clinical and non-clinical environments. Also includes chapters on curriculum design and problem-based learning.*

Mohanna K, Wall D, Chambers R. *Teaching made easy. A manual for health profes-sionals*. Abington: Radcliffe Medical Press; 2004. *Offers clear and relevant advice on a range of teaching issues.*

Swannick T (ed). *Understanding Medical Education: Evidence, Theory and Practice*. Chichester: John Wiley & Sons Ltd.; 2010. *A comprehensive manual addressing all areas of medical education, written by experts in the field.*

Medical education organisations
The Association for the Study of Medical Education (ASME):
www.asme.org.uk
ASME is a membership organisation which aims to provide opportunities for developing medical educators and to promote and disseminate high quality educational research. It publishes two journals: *Medical Education*, containing academic papers, and *The Clinical Teacher*, with a range of articles designed to be accessible to the active practising clinician. ASME holds an annual conference and a variety of smaller conferences and study days. It hosts various interest groups and offers grants and awards for medical education projects.

The Academy of Medical Educators (AOME): www.medicaleducators.org
AOME is a professional organisation supporting those involved in education in medicine, dentistry and veterinary science for the public benefit. It aims to define and promote standards in medical education, and has developed a set of professional standards to allow accreditation as a medical teacher to a national standard. It hosts educational meetings and an on-line journal *Excellence in Medical Education*.

The Association for Medical Education in Europe (AMEE): www.amee.org
AMEE is an international organisation which also holds an annual educational conference (in Europe) and delivers courses on teaching, assessment, simulation, computer-enhanced learning, research and leadership skills. It publishes the journal *Medical Teacher*, a series of education guides and a collection of systematic reviews of evidence on various medical education topics (Best Evidence Medical Education): www.bemecollaboration.org

---

We are now at a point where we must educate our children in what no one knew yesterday, and prepare our schools for what no one knows yet.

Margaret Mead, anthropologist

Appendix **Glossary of assessment tools**

ACAT	Acute Care Assessment Tool (A&E)
ACE	Assessment of Clinical Encounter (psychiatry)
A-CES	Anaesthesia Clinical Evaluation Exercise
DOPS	Directly Observed Procedural Skills
ALMAT	Anaesthesia List Management Assessment Tool
DORPS	Directly Observed Assessment of Radiotherapy Planning Skills
DOST	Directly Observed Assessment of Systemic Therapy Skills
ECE	Evaluation of Clinical/Management Events (pathology)
Mini-ACE	Mini Assessment of Clinical Encounter (psychiatry)
Mini-CEx	Mini Clinical Evaluation Exercise
Mini-IPX	Mini Imaging Interpretation Exercise (radiology)
Mini-PAT	Mini Peer Assessment Tool
MSF	Multi-Source Feedback
OSAT	Objective Structured Assessment of Technical Skills (O&G)
PBA	Procedure Based Assessments (surgery)
PSQ	Patient Survey Questionnaire or Patient Satisfaction Questionnaire
RAD-DOPS	Radiology Direct Observation of Procedural Skills
SAIL	Sheffield Assessment Instrument for Letters
SHEFFPAT	Sheffield Parent Assessment Tool
SPRAT	Sheffield Peer Assessment Tool
TAB	Team Assessment of Behaviour
TO	Team Observation (Obstetrics & Gynaecology)

How to Teach in Clinical Settings, First Edition. Mary Seabrook.
© 2014 John Wiley & Sons, Ltd. Published 2014 by John Wiley & Sons, Ltd.

Index

Academy of Medical Educators
(AOME), 117
accident and emergency
department, 46–7
Acute Care Assessment Tool (ACAT), 68
ad hoc teaching, 100
aids and props, 39, 63. *See also* resources
aims, 31, 42, 45, 52, 54, 94
AMEE (Association for Medical
Education in Europe), 117
AOME (Academy of Medical
Educators), 117
apprenticeship, xi, 1, 6, 23
ASME (Association for the Study of
Medical Education), 117
assessments of performance (AoPs), 68
case-based discussion, 70, 71–2
directly observed procedural
skills, 75–6
glossary of, 118
mini-clinical evaluation
exercise, 73–4
multi-source feedback, 77–8
student's level of experience
and, 94–5
for teaching, 94–6
workplace-based
assessments/supervised learning
events, 67–70 (*See also* feedback)
Association for Medical Education in
Europe (AMEE), 117
Association for the Study of Medical
Education (ASME), 117

bedside teaching, 19, 29–37
bench rounds, 26–8
board rounds, 26–8, 46

case-based discussion (CbD), 69, 70,
71–2, 79
clinic teaching
emergency department and, 46
principles, 38–40
strategies, 40–46
clinical placements, 2–4, 6–10
clinical supervision, 1, 11, 115
colleagues
involvement of, 13–14
teaching of, 64–5, 103
complaints, 96–9
confidence, 1, 2, 50, 103
conscious competence, 57
conscious incompetence, 57
continuing professional
development 110–117
continuity, 8–9
curricula, 5, 10, 40, 111

de-briefing, 30, 33, 34, 41, 54
deliberative practice, 59
difficult consultations, 106
directly observed procedural skills
(DOPS), 68, 69, 75–6
discussion-based assessments, 68

educational supervision, 9, 70, 77, 94, 115
enthusiasm, 9–11, 16, 77, 108, 112
errors, 4, 96–9
European Working Time Directive, 8
evaluation. *See* assessment tools;
self-evaluation
programme/placement
evaluation, 114–15
self-evaluation and, 111–15
expectations, 3–5, 16–17, 50, 69

How to Teach in Clinical Settings, First Edition. Mary Seabrook.
© 2014 John Wiley & Sons, Ltd. Published 2014 by John Wiley & Sons, Ltd.

feedback. *See also* assessment tools
  at bedside, 33–7
  chronological approach to
    feedback, 87
  criteria-based approach to feedback, 87
  errors and, 96
  importance of, 10
  from learners, 113–15
  negative, 81–2
  options for, 85–8
  patient, 35–6
  peer, 35
  principles of, 82
  programme/placement evaluation
    and, 114–15
  strategies, 82–5
  structures for, 85–8
financial support, 92
formative assessments, 67
funding of medical education, 91–3

goal-setting, 10
group learning, 101–2, 105, 107

handover meetings, 26–8
hidden curriculum, 23–4

images interpretation, 47–8
induction, 4–5

Kolb's model of experiential
    learning, 97–8

leadership, 9
learning
  enhancement of, 1–6, 15–17
  in groups, 101–2, 105, 107
  Kolb's model of, 97–8
  of practical skills, 56–60, 105
  quiet/reluctant students and, 104–5
learning climate, 1–6
log books, 6, 51, 109

masters programmes, 116
medical education organisations, 117
mini-clinical evaluation exercise
    (Mini-CEx/Mini-ACE), 68, 69,
    73–4
Mini Peer Assessment Tool
    (Mini-Pat), 68
modelling, 36
multidisciplinary approach, 13–14,
    64–5, 103

multidisciplinary teaching, 13–4, 64–5
multi-source feedback (MSF), 68–9,
    77–8

named clinical supervisor, 9, 70, 94
negative feedback, 81–2

objectives, 5, 7, 29, 54, 70, 79, 97, 100, 111
observational assessments, 68
observational skills, 15, 21–2, 43–5
on-call teaching, 60–62
open/trainee-centred model of
    feedback, 88
operating theatre teaching, 49–55
orientation, 3–5
OSAT (Objective Structured Assessment
    of Technical Skills), 68

patients. *See also* clinic teaching
  bedside teaching and, 19, 29–37
  briefing, 30
  continuity and, 8–9
  difficult consultations and, 106
  education of, 62–4
  involvement of, 11–13
  selecting, 30
peer evaluation, 112
Pendleton's rules, 85
placements, 3, 5–9, 114–15
practical skills teaching, 56–60, 105
professional socialisation, 23–4
procedure-based assessments (PBA), 68
programme evaluation, 114–15
psychiatric ward rounds, 25–6

quiet students, 104–5
questioning, 41–2, 71–4

reflection, 96–8
relatives, 106
reluctant students, 104–5, 108–9
remote teaching, 60–62
resources, 9–10, 39, 63, 79, 115–17
role models, 11, 23–5

Sandwich Model, 85, 87
self-evaluation, 74, 83, 111–15
Service Increment for Teaching
    (SIFT), 91–2
Sheffield Peer Assessment Tool
    (SPRAT), 68
SIFT (service increment for
    teaching), 91–2

skills development, 110–11, 115–16
SLEs. *See* supervised learning events
social support, 3
specimens interpretation, 47–8
student feedback, 113–15
summative assessments, 67
supervised learning events (SLEs)
  background and overview, 67–70
  case-based discussion, 70, 71–2
  directly observed procedural
    skills, 75–6
  effective use of, 69–70
  mini-clinical evaluation
    exercise, 73–4
  multi-source feedback, 77–8
  teaching observation tools, 78–80

TAB (team assessment of behaviour), 68
teaching
  ad hoc, 100
  effectiveness and, 9–11
  groups, 101–2, 105, 107
  level of, 94–5
  multiple students, 107
  observation tool, 79–80
  opportunisitic, 100
  uninterested trainees, 10

principles and strategies, 15–17
quiet/reluctant students and, 104–105,
  108–109
skills development, 110–11,
  115–16
teaching climate, 9–10
team assessment of behaviour
  (TAB), 68
theatre teaching, 49–55
time constraints, 91–3
time pressures, 91–3
training programme director, 1, 99
tuition fees, 92

unconscious competence, 56–7

video evaluation, 112–13

ward rounds
  general principles, 19–21
  psychiatric, 25–6
  strategies, 21–5
work-based learning, 1–2
workplace-based assessments
  (WBAs), 67–70. *See also*
  supervised learning events